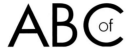

# ABC of

# Lung Cancer

EDITED BY

## Ian Hunt

Thoracic Surgery Fellow
University of Alberta
Edmonton, Canada

## Martin Muers

Consultant Physician
Respiratory Medicine
Leeds General Infirmary
Leeds, UK

## Tom Treasure

Consultant Cardiothoracic Surgeon
Cardiothoracic Centre
Guy's Hospital
London, UK

**WILEY-BLACKWELL**
A John Wiley & Sons, Ltd., Publication

**BMJ|Books**

# Contents

# Contributors

**Jeanette Dickson**
Consultant Clinical Oncologist and Clinical Tutor
Mount Vernon Hospital
Northwood, UK

**Jesme Fox**
Medical Director
The Roy Castle Lung Cancer Foundation
Liverpool, UK

**Fergus Gleeson**
Consultant Radiologist
Churchill Hospital
Oxford, UK

**Jenny Hill**
Director, National Collaborating Centre for Acute Care
National Collaborating Centre for Acute Care
Royal College of Surgeons
London, UK

**Ian Hunt**
Thoracic Surgery Fellow
University of Alberta
Edmonton, Canada

**Patricia Hunt**
Lecturer Practitioner, Palliative Care
The School of Cancer Nursing and Rehabilitation
Royal Marsden Hospital
London, UK

**Sally Moore**
Macmillan Lung Cancer Nurse Specialist
Palliative Care Department
Guy's Hospital
London, UK

**Martin Muers**
Consultant Physician
Respiratory Medicine
Leeds General Infirmary
Leeds, UK

**Richard Neal**
Senior Lecturer in General Practice
Department of General Practice
Cardiff University
Wrexham, UK

**Mike O'Doherty**
Senior Lecturer in Imaging Sciences; Consultant in Nuclear Medicine
Guy's and St Thomas' NHS Trust
London, UK

**Michael Peake**
Consultant Physician, Respiratory Medicine
Glenfield Hospital
Leicester, UK

**Michael Snee**
Consultant Clinical Oncologist
St James' Institute of Oncology
Leeds, UK

**Carol Tan**
Specialist Registrar Thoracic Surgery
Guy's Hospital
London, UK

**Tom Treasure**
Consultant Cardiothoracic Surgeon
Cardiothoracic Centre
Guy's Hospital
London, UK

**Andrew Wilcock**
Macmillan Reader in Palliative Medicine and Medical Oncology
Nottingham City Hospital NHS Trust
Nottingham, UK

**Penella Woll**
Professor of Medical Oncology
University of Sheffield
Sheffield, UK

# Preface

Lung cancer is responsible for 20% of all cancer deaths in the developed world. In the majority of cases it is related to smoking, but despite changes in smoking habits it remains a common cause of cancer death. Prognosis is often poor but cure is possible and when it is not, well considered management may give extension of life and worthwhile palliation.

Managing lung cancer requires a truly multi-disciplinary approach with doctors, nurses, health care professionals from general practice, pulmonary medicine, oncology, radiology, surgery, palliative care and others, playing their part in the care of lung cancer patients.

The *ABC of Lung Cancer* was inspired by the group responsible for the UK lung cancer guidelines (NICE Lung Cancer Guidelines 2005 May 13 Available from http://www.nice.org.uk/ page.aspx?o=244008) and aims to introduce the reader to the important areas of non-small cell lung cancer including its changing epidemiology, the question of screening, current practice in diagnosis and staging, available treatments and palliative care, with separate chapters on small-cell lung cancer and mesothelioma.

The book is written for medical students, doctors in training, specialist nurses, and allied health professionals who may be involved in caring for lung cancer patients. It provides a comprehensive introduction to all aspects of lung cancer care and management.

Ian Hunt
Martin Muers
Tom Treasure

# Acknowledgement

The editors would like to acknowledge the members of the Guideline Development Group of the National Institute for Health and Clinical Excellence (NICE), 2005 Lung Cancer Clinical Guideline, all of whom have assisted in someway, and some of whom have contributed directly, to the publication of the *ABC of Lung Cancer*.

# CHAPTER 1

# Epidemiology, Risk Factors and Prevention

*Martin Muers, Ian Hunt and Jesme Fox*

**OVERVIEW**

- Lung cancer remains an important cause of cancer death throughout the Western world, despite a recent decline.
- The epidemiology of lung cancer in the developing world is likely to increase.
- Smoking remains the single most important cause.
- Other risk factors are recognised.
- Smoking cessation remains the most important step in reducing lung cancer risk.
- Government-supported regulatory control of smoking is also likely to be necessary.

Epidemiology shows that lung cancer is a serious disease, associated with a significant health burden in the UK and in much of the Western world. It is also likely to have a major impact in the developing world, particularly in countries like China where smoking, the number one risk factor for lung cancer, remains unaffected by changes in legislation such as those seen in the USA and Europe (Figure 1.1).

## Epidemiological trends

### The UK perspective
In the UK, lung cancer accounts for 6% of all deaths and roughly one in five of all cancer deaths. Around 38,000 cases are diagnosed, and approximately 33,500 people will die each year. That is more than the number of deaths from breast and bowel cancer combined. Indeed, more women die from lung cancer than breast cancer. Furthermore, only 25% of patients survive the first year following diagnosis, and the five-year survival rate has remained virtually unchanged for 30 years at approximately 7%.

However, with changing perceptions of smoking in the UK there has been a large reduction in smoking amongst men in the last 50 years, from a peak national consumption of about 12 cigarettes per male per day in 1945 to 4.6 per day by 1992. The incidence of lung cancer in men has declined correspondingly; from 80–120

*ABC of Lung Cancer.* Edited by I. Hunt, M. Muers and T. Treasure. © 2009 Blackwell Publishing, ISBN: 978-1-4051-4652-4.

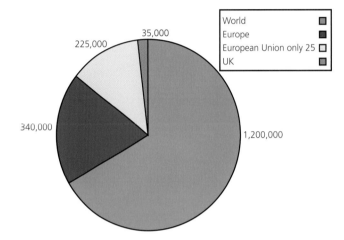

**Figure 1.1** The global burden of lung cancer in terms of cases per year.

per 100,000 in 1962 to 70–100 per 100,000 by 2002 (Figures 1.2 and 1.3).

In men at least, the UK incidence rates are comparable to many other European countries. By contrast, lung cancer death rates in women are not yet falling universally across all age cohorts, as their peak tobacco consumption occurred in 1974. Consumption has now fallen by about 50%, but as corresponding lung cancer mortality rates lag behind changes in smoking habits the mortality rate amongst women continues to rise (Figure 1.3). In fact, the UK has one of the highest incidence rates of any country in Europe (Box 1.1).

As well as a change in trends amongst men and women, lung cancer is now rare in individuals below the age of 40. The average age at presentation is currently approximately 75 years.

Lung cancer is 2–3 times more common in deprived areas compared to affluent regions of the country. As such, there is considerable regional variation in lung cancer mortality rates in the UK. The highest rates are found in Scotland and northern England, and reflect regional smoking patterns. This has major implications for prevention strategies.

### An international perspective
Many of the epidemiological trends seen in the UK are seen in other Western countries, particularly in Europe. There are around 243,000 deaths from lung cancer each year in European Union (EU)

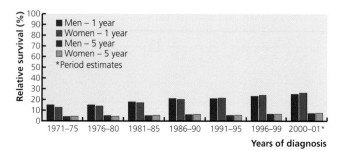

**Figure 1.2** Relative survival rates for lung cancer in England and Wales from 1971 to 2001. (Reproduced with permission from Toms 2004.)

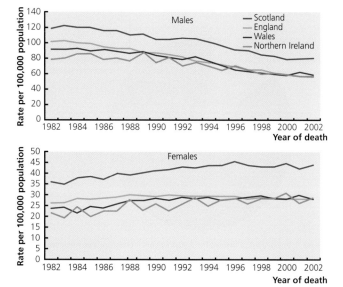

**Figure 1.3** European age-standardised mortality rates for lung cancer in England, Wales, Scotland and Northern Ireland from 1982 to 2002. (Reproduced with permission from Toms 2004.)

---

Box 1.1 **Lung cancer and gender**

In the UK lung cancer amongst men has declined with the reduction in men smoking, but in women lung cancer rates continue to rise as proportionally more women smoke. More women die from lung cancer than breast cancer.

---

countries (188,000 in men and 55,000 in women). For men there has been a small decrease in the number of deaths from lung cancer since a peak in the early 1980s. However, lung cancer remains the biggest cancer killer, accounting for around 50 deaths per 100,000 men in 1995. However, in women lung cancer continues its gradual rise, resulting in about 22 deaths per 100,000 inhabitants in 1996. The highest male lung cancer incidence and mortality rates are found in Hungary, Poland and Belgium, with the lowest rates in Sweden and Portugal. Amongst females the highest lung cancer incidence and mortality rates are found in Denmark,

Hungary and the UK, whilst the lowest are in Spain, Portugal and Malta (Figure 1.4).

In the USA lung cancer is the primary cancer killer in both men and women; during 2006 there were an estimated 174,470 new cases diagnosed. In the USA men have higher rates of lung cancer than females. In 2003, 78.5 per 100,000 men compared to 51.3 per 100,000 women were diagnosed with the disease. However, lung cancer incidence rates have been decreasing significantly among men whilst the rate has been stable since 1998 in women, after a long period of increases. In 1987, it surpassed breast cancer to become the leading cause of cancer deaths in women. The age-adjusted death rate in the black population was 12% greater than the rate in the white population. Similar regional variations among affluent and deprived areas are seen in the USA.

Beyond the West, in countries of the developing world and the 'boom' economies of the Far East and the Indian sub-continent, lung cancer rates remain low compared to those seen in the USA and Europe. However, the epidemiology of lung cancer is likely to change dramatically in the next 30 years in these countries unless curbs are placed on smoking.

The geographical differences seen represent the different stages of the worldwide tobacco epidemic. Although lung cancer incidence and mortality is declining slowly in most countries in Western Europe, in the USA and Australasia, and particularly in Asia, the increase in smoking habits means that sadly world lung cancer mortality is certain to rise from its current level of approximately one million deaths per annum in the 21st century.

## Smoking

The classic early epidemiological study by Doll and Hill in 1950 was followed by the 'doctors' study in which the smoking patterns and health outcome of 20,000 British doctors were followed for 50 years – a unique achievement (Figure 1.5). This study and others have demonstrated unequivocally that: smoking causes lung cancer; the risks are proportional to the dose; quitting reduces that risk; but that even after quitting additional risks remain for more than 40 years (Figure 1.6).

The lifetime risk of a continuing smoker developing lung cancer is approximately 1 in 15, whereas for a lifelong non-smoker it is 1 in 200–300. If people quit at 50 years of age they reduce their lifetime risk to approximately 1 in 30. One consequence of this is that the proportion of lung cancer occurring in ex rather than current smokers in the UK is increasing, and is now at about 50%.

There is no such thing as a 'safe cigarette'. Smokers become very proficient at controlling their preferred nicotine dose. For example, they can achieve a quick increase in levels by taking several deep inhalations when anxious or can opt for lower sustained levels when bored. The increasing use of low-tar cigarettes and filters may be responsible for the rise in frequency of adenocarcinoma, as the smoke is inhaled further out into the lung as the smoker tends to inhale more deeply. As a proportion of all cancers, this particular form has increased from about 15 to 30% in the last 20 years. The risk of lung cancer for long-term pipe smokers and the habitual cigar smoker is lower, but these forms of smoking do also cause cancer.

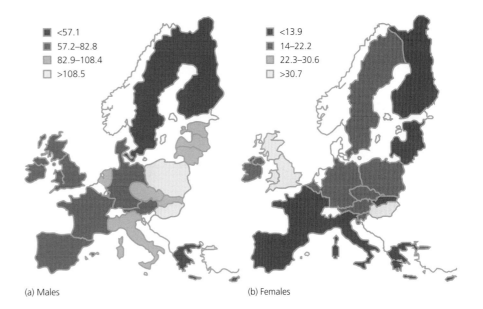

Figure 1.4 legend:

Left map:
- <57.1
- 57.2–82.8
- 82.9–108.4
- >108.5

Right map:
- <13.9
- 14–22.2
- 22.3–30.6
- >30.7

(a) Males          (b) Females

**Figure 1.4** Two maps of Europe highlighting the difference in cancer incidence and mortality between males and females.

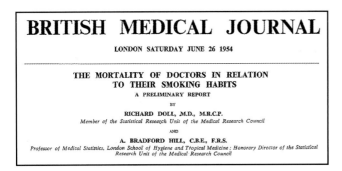

**Figure 1.5** The original 'headline' that appeared in the British Medical Journal in 1954 following Doll and Hill's study.

## Risk factors additional to active tobacco smoking

The rates of spontaneous lung cancer increase with age and account for about 10% of all forms. Some lung cancers never seem to be associated with tobacco. An example is bronchoalveolar-cell carcinoma (BAC), which mimics a chronic unresolving pneumonia. These tumours spread within the lung segment or lobe and the majority do not metastasise (Table 1.1).

The most important additional risk factors are passive smoking and asbestos. There is strong epidemiological evidence that the relative risk to long-term passive smokers is 20–30% above baseline for a spouse or partner, and higher for workplace exposure, and that this causes about 600 lung cancer deaths yearly in the UK. This underpins the banning and restriction of smoking in the workplace and enclosed public places, which is already in force in several American states, some European countries, Scotland and, more recently, England.

People with symptomatic pulmonary asbestosis secondary to occupational exposure, have a 500% increase in their risk of lung cancer. There is a debate as to whether this risk is confined to persons with asbestosis, or whether asbestos itself is a carcinogen. Although

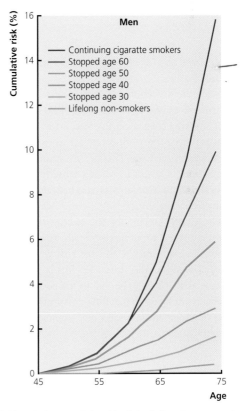

**Figure 1.6** The relative cumulative risk of death from lung cancer in men in the UK, and the effects of stopping smoking at different ages on this risk. (Reproduced with permission from Peto *et al.* 2000.)

unresolved it is likely that asbestos does increase the risk on its own and in proportion to the intensity and duration of exposure.

Radon is a naturally occurring radioactive gas that leaches out of granite. Therefore, people living in houses built upon granite are at an increased risk. This is of considerable importance in countries

**Table 1.1** Lung cancer risk factors other than cigarette smoking.

| Factor | Relative risk |
| --- | --- |
| Environmental tobacco smoke | 1.2 |
| Asbestos (risk proportional to dose) | 1.0–5.0 |
| Radon gas (granite rock) | 1.2 |
| Diesel fumes (occupational) | 1.3 |
| Silicosis | 2.5–3.2 |
| Family history (especially women) <50 yr | 2–4 (unconfirmed) |
| Gender (women at greater risk) | 1.2–1.7 |
| Chronic obstructive pulmonary disease | 2.7–5.0 |

---

**Box 1.2 Methods for reducing lung cancer mortality**

- Primary prevention: stopping children starting
- Secondary prevention: 'quit' programmes
- Chemo prevention: no evidence of benefit yet
- Screening: trials in progress
- Reducing interval between first symptom and treatment: cancer standards
- Better treatments: ongoing clinical research

---

**Box 1.3 Recommendations for smoking cessation programmes in primary care**

- Ask about smoking at every opportunity
- Advise all smokers to stop
- Assist the smoker to stop
- Arrange follow-up
- Assistance:
  - set quit date
  - review past attempts
  - warn about symptoms
  - tell family and friends
  - discuss alcohol consumption
  - provide nicotine replacement therapy

Adapted with permission from Raw *et al.* 1998.

---

**Box 1.4 Key provisions in the Framework Convention on Tobacco Control (FCTC)**

- Enact comprehensive bans on tobacco advertising, promotion and sponsorship.
- Obligate the placement of rotating health warnings on tobacco packaging to cover at least 30% of the principal display areas.
- Ban the use of misleading terms such as 'light' and 'mild'.
- Protect citizens from exposure to tobacco smoke in workplaces, on public transport and in indoor public areas.
- Combat smuggling.
- Increase tobacco taxes.

---

such as Sweden, and to a lesser extent in the south-west of the UK and in Wales.

Women are more susceptible to lung disease, including both chronic obstructive pulmonary disease (COPD) and lung cancer, as a result of smoking than men; the reason for this is unknown. This fact makes it even more important for us to develop primary prevention strategies that are effective in young women. Lung cancer is currently the fastest increasing cause of cancer death in women, yet in the UK 38% of females aged between 20 and 24 years are regular smokers.

People with COPD are at an increased risk of developing lung cancer compared to others with an equivalent smoking history but normal spirometry, and the risk is roughly proportional to COPD severity. The reason for this is unknown. It has been hypothesised that it may be due to the additional effects of a separate tobacco-induced airway inflammation or, less plausibly, to the effects of altered airflow rates on carcinogen deposition in peripheral lung tissue.

## Prevention

Prevention is by far the most effective way by which we could reduce lung cancer mortality (Box 1.2). However, primary prevention is weak in the UK: by the age of 15, one in every four children is a regular smoker and it is estimated that 450 children start smoking every day. It is at this time that nicotine addiction develops.

Altering this pattern of behaviour will be difficult. It will probably need a combination of social and pricing policies and social pressures. Government action taken in Europe and the USA includes cigarette and tobacco packet health warnings, banning tobacco advertisements in all media, health education and, most recently, a ban on smoking in all public places. Parental habits and peer pressure appear to be the two driving factors in most cases and are far less susceptible to alteration.

Nicotine is highly addictive. Mark Twain famously said 'quitting smoking is the easiest thing in the world to do; I have done it several times.' Thus, although more than 70% of smokers would like to quit, long-term quit rates remain low. Simple unequivocal advice by a doctor produces a quit rate of 1–3%. If nicotine replacement therapy and support are added, the quit rate rises to about 6–8%. However, this action tends to be concentrated on adults over the age of 50. Because young people consult their physicians less often, the impact on younger smokers is less. Quit programmes (Box 1.3) cost £800 per life-year saved (1998 data); lung cancer chemotherapy is about 25 times as expensive.

International agencies both in the EU and worldwide, such as the World Health Organisation (WHO), are attempting to combat the menace of the active promotion of cigarette smoking by the large multinational tobacco companies. The WHO Framework Convention on Tobacco Control (FCTC) is an example of this action (Box 1.4). It remains to be seen whether concerted regulatory action by the world's governments will be powerful enough to halt the trend of increased smoking in developing countries, which threatens to engulf fledgling health services and result in a huge burden of tobacco-related diseases in the second half of the 21st century and beyond.

## Further reading

Britton J, ed. *ABC of Smoking Cessation*. BMJ Books, London, 2004.

Muer M. Lung cancer. *Medicine* 2003; **31**(11): 28–37.

Peto R, Darby S, Deo H, Silcocks P, Whitley E & Doll R. Smoking, smoking cessation, and lung cancer in the UK since 1950: combination of national statistics with two case-control studies. *British Medical Journal* 2000; **321**: 323–329.

Raw M, McNeill A & West R. Smoking cessation guidelines for health professionals. *Thorax* 1998; **53**: S5.

Royal College of Physicians. *Nicotine Addition in Britain: A Report of the Tobacco Advisory Group of the Royal College of Physicians*. RCP, London, 2000.

Toms JR, ed. *CancerStats Monograph 2004*. Cancer Research UK, London, 2004.

# CHAPTER 2

# Symptoms and Assessment

*Richard Neal and Martin Muers*

## OVERVIEW

- Detection of lung cancer relies on the recognition of symptoms and signs, which may be vague and non-specific.
- The common clinical manifestations of lung cancer reflect whether they arise from the primary tumour, from local intrathoracic or extrathoracic metastatic spread of the tumour, or are general systemic symptoms.
- Urgent referral guidelines aim to help the healthcare professional in the case of patients at risk of lung cancer presenting with new or persistent symptoms.
- Detection of early-stage lung cancer is associated with an improved outcome.

Box 2.1 **Lung cancer and clinical presentation**

Cough is the commonest presenting symptom in patients with lung cancer; others may have breathlessness and, less commonly, chest pain. Haemoptysis is worrying and may suggest locally advanced disease.

Lung cancer is responsible for nearly one in five of all cancer deaths in the UK and is the most common cause of cancer death in both men and women. As there are no early diagnostic tests or effective screening programme currently, most patients present with symptoms. Early diagnosis both in primary and secondary care depends on history and clinical examination, and subsequent referral for chest X-ray (CXR) and/or a specialist opinion. Patients diagnosed with earlier-stage cancer are more likely to have a curable tumour.

## Opportunistically identifying patients at risk

Most lung cancers occur over the age of 60, the incidence increasing with age, and more men are affected than women. Symptoms and any signs are typically vague and non-specific, often in the context of long-standing problems such as a 'smokers cough' (Box 2.1). If there are any suspicious respiratory symptoms, a history of cigarette smoking is the best indicator of likelihood of lung cancer: 90% of cases are smokers or ex-smokers (Figure 2.1). The risk is cumulative, and is most strongly related to the duration and the amount of tobacco smoked. A pack-year calculation is helpful (20 cigarettes per day for a year being a pack-year) and

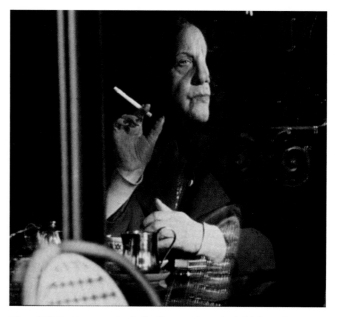

**Figure 2.1** Smoking remains by far the most important risk factor for lung cancer.

passive smoking is also relevant (Box 2.2). Occupational factors are also important; for example, a history of exposure to asbestos. In addition, there is an increased risk associated with a family history of lung cancer and previous head and neck cancer.

## Presenting symptoms

Patients may present with pulmonary symptoms as a result of either the primary tumour or local intrathoracic spread, symptoms

*ABC of Lung Cancer.* Edited by I. Hunt, M. Muers and T. Treasure. © 2009 Blackwell Publishing, ISBN: 978-1-4051-4652-4.

**Table 2.1** Common lung cancer manifestations (Adapted with permission from Collins *et al.* 2007).

| Primary tumour | Intrathoracic spread | Extrathoracic spread |
| --- | --- | --- |
| Cough | Chest wall invasion | Bone pain, fracture |
| Dyspnoea | Oesophageal symptoms | Confusion, personality change |
| Chest discomfort | Horner syndrome | Elevated alkaline phosphatase level |
| Haemoptysis | | Focal neurological deficits |
| | Pancoast's tumour | Headache |
| | Phrenic nerve paralysis | Nausea, vomiting |
| | Pleural effusion | Palpable lymphadenopathy |
| | Recurrent laryngeal nerve paralysis | Seizures |
| | Superior vena cava obstruction | Weakness |
| | | Weight loss |

**Table 2.2** Range of frequency of initial symptoms and signs of lung cancer (Reproduced with permission from Beckles *et al.* 2003).

| Symptoms and signs | Range of frequency (%) |
| --- | --- |
| Cough | 8–75 |
| Weight loss | 0–68 |
| Dyspnoea | 3–60 |
| Chest pain | 20–49 |
| Haemoptysis | 6–35 |
| Bone pain | 6–25 |
| Clubbing | 0–20 |
| Fever | 0–20 |
| Weakness | 0–10 |
| Superior vena cava obstruction (SVCO) | 0–4 |
| Dysphagia | 0–2 |
| Wheezing and stridor | 0–2 |

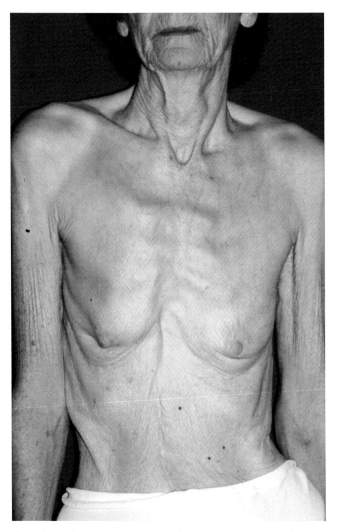

**Figure 2.2** Unheralded significant loss of weight may be caused by lung cancer, but other causes (and cancers) must first be excluded.

related to extrathoracic spread or metastases, and more general systemic symptoms of ill health (Table 2.1). Over three quarters of patients with lung cancer will present with a cough, particularly if it has changed in character or become persistent. Some patients complain of dyspnoea or breathlessness and may have chest pain of some kind. Haemoptysis is often a symptom of more extensive disease, as is hoarseness (due to damage to the recurrent laryngeal nerve caused by the tumour). Symptoms of metastatic disease include bone pain (pathological fractures) and fits, confusion or headache (cerebral metastases). These may sometimes be the predominant presenting symptoms (Table 2.2). Symptoms of general ill health including weight loss, fatigue and anorexia are non-specific, relatively common presenting symptoms (Figure 2.2). Haemoptysis, dyspnoea and abnormal spirometry remained independently associated with lung cancer after exclusion of symptoms reported in the six months prior to diagnosis.

## Clinical examination

Many of the symptoms, signs and clinical findings in suspected lung cancer are indistinguishable from those of other lung

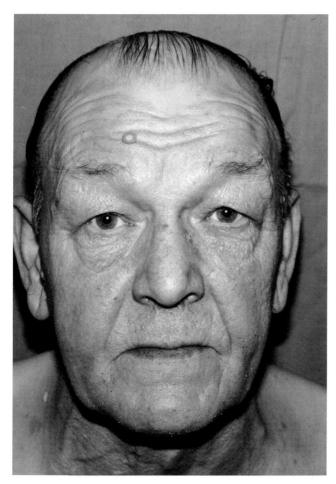

**Figure 2.3** A patient with distended neck veins suggestive of superior vena cava obstruction associated with a central tumour or enlarged mediastinal lymph nodes.

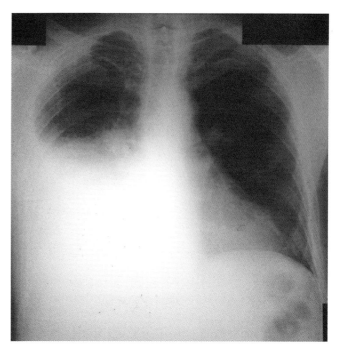

**Figure 2.4** An abnormal chest X-ray (CXR) with large right pleural effusion.

pathologies, in particular chronic obstructive pulmonary disease (COPD) with which the cancer may co-exist. The difficulty the clinician faces is identifying patients most likely to have lung cancer without carrying out a large number of chest radiographs. There is no easy way of doing this. Being vigilant for those most at risk, particularly smokers and ex-smokers, for example those that present with new symptoms that have lasted for more than three weeks or with changes in existing symptoms, and a low threshold of suspicion in such patients is essential.

There may be breathlessness at rest or upon minimal exertion, and noisy laboured breathing. There may be localizing signs in the chest, e.g. signs of lobar collapse, consolidation or a unilateral pleural effusion. More specific signs include supraclavicular lymphadenopathy, finger clubbing and signs of superior vena cava obstruction – a swollen neck or face, suffused conjunctivae, stridor or a persistent haemoptysis or hoarseness (Figure 2.3). Patients with lung cancer may be cachectic, be pale or clinically anaemic, and appear wasted or generally unwell. Signs of metastatic disease

might include hepatomegaly, skin metastases or evidence of raised intracranial pressure.

Guidance on referral for patients with symptoms and signs of suspected lung cancer is now readily available (see Chapter 3) and has been published by the National Institute of Health and Clinical Excellence (NICE 2005).

## Investigations

### Chest radiography

CXR is the initial investigation of choice for most patients with a clinical possibility of lung cancer. Most nodules greater than 1 cm in diameter will be identified on a CXR and, if identified in a patient at risk, will raise a strong possibility of lung cancer. Others may cause collapse/consolidation or a unilateral pleural effusion (Figure 2.4); these will be detected by a CXR, usually with a radiologist recommendation for a further CXR or other radiology within a period of three weeks to see if there is a specific underlying cause, or a recommendation for an urgent referral. However, some small cancers may not be detected by a single CXR and, in the face of ongoing suspicious symptoms and a normal CXR, referral to a chest physician or for a further CXR within a period of a few weeks is advised.

### Blood tests, sputum and other radiology

While waiting for the CXR report (which, depending on local provision may take between one and two weeks to receive in primary care) it is common practice to undertake simple blood and other investigations. These could include a full blood count (which may show anaemia), liver function tests (which may be

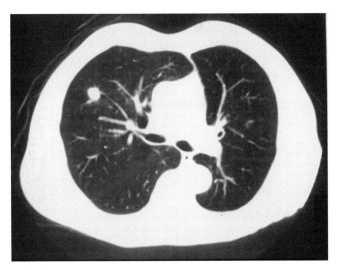

**Figure 2.5** A computed tomography (CT) scan showing nodular mass in right lung field.

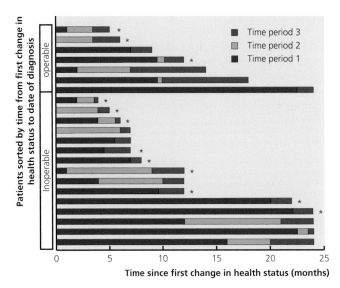

**Figure 2.6** Delays between the time from first change in health status to diagnosis and where they occur. Time period 1 (red) is the time from first recalled change in health status to onset of the symptom that prompted a patient's visit to a general practitioner or other service. Time period 2 (green) is the time from the onset of the symptom to the first visit to the general practitioner (GP) or other service. Time period 3 (blue) is the time from the visit to the GP to the date of diagnosis.

abnormal in the presence of liver metastases), plasma viscosity or erythrocyte sedimentation rate (which may be raised in malignancy), and serum calcium (which may be raised if there are bone metastases or in squamous carcinoma). Sputum cytology is rarely undertaken, although it is sometimes indicated if the patient is not thought likely to be able to tolerate or accept a bronchoscopy or similar. Computed tomography (CT) scanning or other imaging is usually reserved for staging investigations if needed and is not routinely undertaken at a prediagnostic stage, unless presenting symptoms are atypical or it is recommended by a reporting radiologist (Figure 2.5). Spirometry may show airflow obstruction, and the risk of lung cancer is raised in patients with COPD.

## Diagnostic pathways

Whilst the majority of patients with lung cancer are diagnosed following referrals from primary care (whether urgent or non-urgent), many patients are diagnosed following an emergency admission or whilst already in hospital. A small number are found opportunistically following a CXR for an unrelated reason. The reasons for these different diagnostic pathways include the nature and severity of symptoms and their interpretation by the patient, and the response of general practitioners to the symptoms. The important issue is that each patient is diagnosed at as early a stage as possible, rather than how they are diagnosed. Patients presenting directly to secondary care rather than through primary care are likely to have less overall delay; however, this is probably because of more advanced disease at initial symptom presentation.

A patient referred to a hospital outpatient clinic by their general practitioner is most likely to see a consultant respiratory physician. The pattern of subsequent investigations may vary, but an example of good practice is for a patient to be offered a choice of days to attend for a diagnostic CT scan with contrast, followed on the

same day by either a fibreoptic bronchoscopy or a transthoracic fine-needle biopsy, depending upon the radiographic findings. At this time the patient will meet a nurse specialist for the first time. Further investigations may follow and the patient is likely to be discussed by the multidisciplinary team (MDT; see Chapter 3). Following this meeting, the patient should expect in most cases to be told definitively what the diagnosis is, and what the plan is for treatment or further investigation.

## Diagnostic delays

The delay from the first change in health status to diagnosis of lung cancer in the UK did stand at a mean of 88 days (median 38 days); however, with the implementation of referral guidelines and waiting time initiatives this is likely to have fallen (Figure 2.6). Most delays occur prior to patients getting to hospital. About two-thirds of the delay is 'patient delay'; i.e. when patients are symptomatic but have yet to present symptoms in primary care or elsewhere. This can occur when, for example, patients fail to recognize the significance of a symptom such as prolonged cough. Internationally, there is little difference in the time from a patient's first perception of the change in health status to the time when they seek medical advice. This is the predominant delay, and in general terms delays subsequently are dependent on health systems. About one-third of the delay is primary care delay; i.e. from when symptoms are presented to primary care to referral to secondary care. This can occur for example when patients present with non-respiratory symptoms such as shoulder pain. No significant sociodemographic factors are relevant for lung cancer diagnostic delays.

## Further reading

Beckles MA, Spiro SG, Colice GL & Rudd RM. Initial evaluation of the patient with lung cancer: symptoms, signs, laboratory tests, and paraneoplastic syndromes. *Chest* 2003; **123**(suppl. 1): 97S–104S.

Collins LG, Haines C, Perkel R & Enck RE. Lung cancer: diagnosis and management. *American Family Physician* 2007; **75**: 56–63.

Hamilton WT, Peters TJ, Round AP & Sharp DJ. What are the clinical features of lung cancer before the diagnosis is made? A population-based case-control study. *Thorax* 2005; **60**(12): 1059–1065.

NICE. *Referral Guidelines for Suspected Cancer.* NICE Clinical Guideline No. 27. National Institute for Health & Clinical Excellence, London 2005: http://www.nice.org.uk.

Toms JR, ed. *CancerStats Monograph 2004.* Cancer Research UK, London, 2004.

# CHAPTER 3

# Service Organisation and Guidelines for Referral

*Michael Peake, Richard Neal and Andrew Wilcock*

## OVERVIEW

- Clinical guidelines aim to help the referring healthcare professional in the case of patients with suspected lung cancer.
- Whenever there is a suspicion of lung cancer the primary care physician should have ready access to chest clinic referral.
- Primary care physicians need immediate access to chest radiography.
- There should be a policy in place regarding whether a clinic appointment should be triggered by discovery of an abnormal chest radiograph or should be requested by the primary care physician.
- The diagnosis, staging and management of all patients with lung cancer should be discussed in a meeting of a multidisciplinary team (MDT).

Lung cancer is now the commonest solid tumour in the developed world. Whatever the basis of healthcare provision, there have to be agreed standards of care by the profession and routes of access for the patients.

## The diagnostic pathway

### Referral and rapid access clinics

At present the majority of patients with lung cancer (80–90%) are first seen for treatment of the disease when it is beyond hope of cure with available treatments. Earlier diagnosis is one obvious way in which this might be improved and there is guidance on how this might be achieved (Table 3.1). However, there is little high-level evidence to support such guidance and it is largely based on the consensus of expert opinion.

Nevertheless, since most non-small cell lung cancers (NSCLC) are at some point localised and later are disseminated, there are compelling reasons to make the diagnosis as early as possible. The goal is to provide both rapid access and rapid diagnosis for patients with a suspected diagnosis of cancer. Most acute hospitals now run dedicated rapid access lung cancer clinics with referral being to the service rather than to a named consultant.

## Guidance on referring patients with suspected lung cancer

The UK urgent cancer referral guidance was recently revised following its introduction in 2000. The guidance published by NICE in 2005 is based upon the best evidence currently available (see Box 3.1). However, currently only 23% of patients with lung cancer are diagnosed in this manner and only 42% of urgent referrals are diagnosed with lung cancer. Whilst these figures compare favourably with other cancers, they are only likely to improve once the evidence base on which the guidance is based is improved, and the guidance becomes more widely implemented. There is a need for a greater understanding of the clinical epidemiology of symptoms, and randomised controlled trials for implementation (Box 3.2).

## Investigations in primary care

Any of the most complex investigations in a patient presenting with a suspicion of lung cancer can be requested in primary care, but typically the first investigation requested is the chest X-ray (CXR). The CXR is almost always abnormal by the time a patient with lung cancer has symptoms (although it is important to remember that a normal X-ray does not exclude the diagnosis) and so is a key step in the early part of the diagnostic pathway. Clinicians in primary care should therefore have easy access to this service.

The next question is how should the discovery of abnormalities be handled? If it automatically triggers a chest clinic referral this may alarm the patient while the referring general practitioner is unaware of the findings. On the other hand, if the original intention was to find any abnormalities in order to act upon them, returning a written report to the referring family doctor may waste precious time in pursuing a cancer. There will be different solutions in different healthcare systems. Clearly there is a need for clearly defined pathways.

## Investigations in secondary care

A staging computed tomography (CT) scan of the thorax and upper abdomen should come before bronchoscopy and may be arranged prior to the first visit to clinic. This may speed up the diagnostic process and allows for a much more informed discussion to

*ABC of Lung Cancer.* Edited by I. Hunt, M. Muers and T. Treasure. © 2009 Blackwell Publishing, ISBN: 978-1-4051-4652-4.

**Table 3.1** Summary of published UK and international clinical guidelines for lung cancer.

| Date | Source | Country | Title | Reference |
|---|---|---|---|---|
| 1998 | The Lung Cancer Working Party of the British Thoracic Society Standards of Care Committee | UK | Recommendations to Respiratory Physicians for Organising the Care of Patients with Lung Cancer | *Thorax* 1998; **53**: (suppl I): S1–81 www.brit-thoracic.org.uk |
| 2001 | British Thoracic Society and Society of Cardiothoracic Surgeons of Great Britain and Ireland Working Party | UK | Guideline for the Selection of Patients with Lung Cancer for Surgery | *Thorax* 2001; **56**: 89–108 www.brit-thoracic.org.uk |
| 2003 | French National Federation of Cancer Centres (FNCLCC) | France | Guidelines on Non-Small Cell Lung Cancer | www.fnclcc.fr |
| 2005 | Scottish Intercollegiate Guidelines Network | Scotland | Management of Patients with Lung Cancer | www.sign.ac.uk |
| 2005 | National Institute for Clinical Excellence | England | The Diagnosis and Treatment of Lung Cancer | www.nice.org.uk |
| 2007 | American College of Chest Physicians (ACCP) | USA | Diagnosis and Management of Lung Cancer: ACCP Evidence-Based Clinical Practice Guidelines (2nd Edition) | *Chest* 2007; **132** (suppl 3): 1S–19 www.chestnet.org |
| 2008 | US National Comprehensive Cancer Network (NCCN) | USA | Guidelines on Non-Small Cell Lung Cancer | www.nccn.org |

---

Box 3.1 **Role of clinical guidelines**

Guidelines aim to improve patient care through agreed standards of practice based on assessment of current body of evidence.

---

take place between the hospital specialist and the patient (and their carers) at their first visit.

The potential complexity of the diagnostic and staging process combined with the fact that many lung cancer patients have significant comorbidities means that there is a need for careful planning of the pathway and support for patients over this difficult time. Guidance is now available on approaching the diagnosis of suspected lung cancer (see Figure 3.1).

## Positron emission tomography

Positron emission tomography (PET) scanning using 18F-fluorodeoxyglucose (FDG) as the tracer is now well established as of value in the staging and diagnosis of lung cancer (see Chapter 4). In the new generation of scanners it is always in combination with CT scanning (PET-CT; Box 3.3).

## Multidisciplinary teams

All lung cancer patients should be reviewed in a meeting of a multidisciplinary team (MDT). The team should convene at least weekly in a multidisciplinary meeting (MDM; Figure 3.2). The main rationale for such teams and meetings is to ensure that all patients have their diagnosis, stage and management plan discussed by a team of specialists covering all of the relevant disciplines. It is no longer acceptable for one particular speciality to act as 'gatekeeper' to referral for consideration of radical therapies. In the case of lung cancer however, the respiratory physician makes an appropriate and even-handed chair – a high proportion of patients come through the chest clinics and the respiratory physician does not deliver the

---

Box 3.2 **Referral guidelines when lung cancer is suspected**

- A patient who presents with symptoms suggestive of lung cancer should be referred to a team specializing in the management of lung cancer, depending upon local circumstances.
- An urgent referral for a CXR should be made when a patient presents with haemoptysis, or any of the following unexplained persistent (that is, lasting more than three weeks) symptoms and signs:
  - chest and/or shoulder pain;
  - dyspnoea;
  - weight loss;
  - chest signs;
  - hoarseness;
  - finger clubbing;
  - cervical and/or supraclavicular lymphadenopathy;
  - cough with or without any of the above; or
  - features suggestive of metastasis from a lung cancer (e.g. brain, bone, liver, skin).
- An urgent referral should be for any of the following:
  - persistent haemoptysis in smokers or ex-smokers who are aged 40 years or over; or
  - a CXR suggestive of lung cancer (including pleural effusion and slowly resolving consolidation).
- Immediate referral should be considered for the following:
  - signs of superior vena caval obstruction (swelling of the face and/or neck with fixed elevation of jugular venous pressure); or
  - stridor.
- Patients in the following categories have a higher risk of developing lung cancer:
  - are current or ex-smokers;
  - have smoking-related COPD;
  - have been exposed to asbestos; or
  - have had a previous history of cancer (especially head and neck).

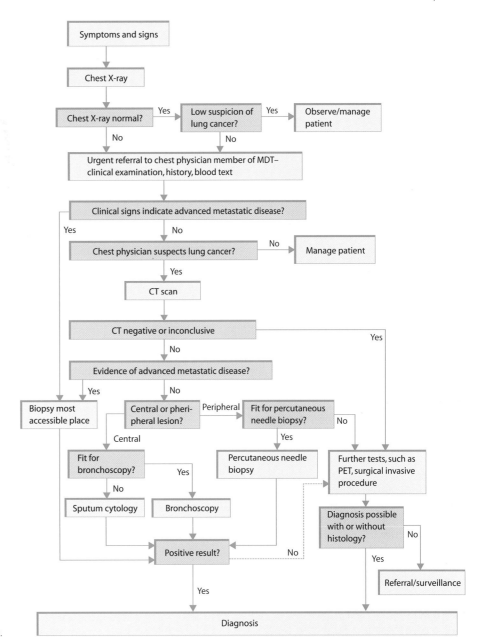

**Figure 3.1** Diagnosis of lung cancer. CT, computed tomography; MDT, multidisciplinary team; PET, positron emission tomography. (Reproduced with permission from NICE 2005).

Box 3.3 **How positron emission tomography (PET) works**

PET is a non-invasive, diagnostic investigation that finds information about the activity of different parts of the body. Those parts of the body that are the most active need energy, and the energy that it uses includes glucose. A PET scan can use a specially created substance that the body thinks is glucose and takes up into the cells. This substance is called a 'tracer', and it is almost exactly like glucose, but has a small radioactive part attached or 'tagged' to it. The images are based on the detection of radiation from the emission of positrons (positively charged electrons) that are made as the radioactive tracer is broken down inside your body. The subsequent images created are used to evaluate a variety of diseases, with the most common use being whole-body imaging of cancer. The most commonly used glucose-based radioactive tracer in investigating lung cancer is fluorodeoxyglucose (FDG).

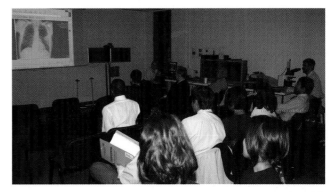

**Figure 3.2** The multidisciplinary team (MDT) meeting.

Box 3.4 **Ideal members of lung cancer multidisciplinary teams**

**'Core' clinical members**
- Respiratory physician
- Thoracic radiologist
- Pathologist
- Thoracic surgeon
- Medical oncologist
- Clinical oncologist
- Palliative care physician
- Clinical nurse specialists (including research nurse)

**Administrative members**
- MDT coordinator
- Audit coordinator
- Patient tracker

**'Associate' clinical members**
- Clinical librarian
- Clinical psychologist
- Social worker
- Occupational therapist
- Physiotherapist
- Dietician
- Bereavement officer

Box 3.5 **Role of particular 'core' members of the MDT**

- **Radiology:** accurate staging can be very difficult in this disease and requires high quality radiology. This can be difficult in smaller hospitals where small numbers of more general radiologists have, of necessity, to cover a range of diseases.
- **Thoracic surgery:** the main means of cure is surgical resection. The presence of a thoracic surgeon with particular expertise in the staging and treatment of lung cancer is essential to ensure that patients with potentially curable disease are not overlooked.
- **Oncology:** modern cancer care demands the presence of both medical and radiation oncologists.

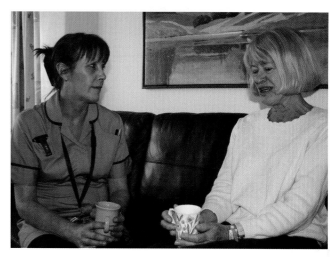

Figure 3.3 A patient with a community cancer nurse specialist.

Box 3.6 **Role of the specialist cancer nurse**

- **Patient's key worker:** ensuring the patient is given information they need and want at the time they would like it.
- **Indirect patient care:** liaison between hospital and the patient, at the multidisciplinary team (MDT) discussions, with other team members within the hospital and in the community, including specialized units such as hospices.
- **Providing emotional support:** helping the patient and family cope by answering questions and dealing with fears associated with illness.
- **Providing information:** available to support and advice patients about their investigations, results, diagnosis and treatment.
- **Support through the treatment pathway:** facilitates the process by being a point of contact for the different specialists and often for hospitals involved in treating the patient.
- **Deal with specific clinical problems:** identify, assess and aid in management decisions for symptoms such as pain or breathlessness.

main target therapies and should have no conflict of interests in the major management decisions.

The members of a lung cancer MDT are listed in Box 3.4. Not all need to be present throughout every meeting. However, it could be argued that all patients should be reviewed by at least radiology, thoracic surgery and oncology (see Box 3.5). To date, there is little data published in peer-reviewed journals objectively demonstrating improved outcomes as a result of MDT working.

## Follow-up

One of the problems of multidisciplinary management is that follow-up after diagnosis and treatment can be less clear-cut. Joint surveillance by both the treating clinician and a respiratory physician is probably ideal, since many patients have ongoing significant respiratory problems such as pleural effusions and chronic obstructive pulmonary disease (COPD). Nurse-led follow up can be effective and safe. There is concern that some patients not followed up with oncological input may miss out on second-line therapies, which could improve both symptoms and survival. There

is also scope for a much-improved liaison between hospital-based services and those in the community.

## Lung cancer nurse specialist

Palliative care works best if there is a named 'key worker' and specialist nurse input can greatly aid timely and appropriate supportive care. Lung cancer nurse specialists can act as the key worker and are in the best position to provide the link between hospital and community healthcare (Figure 3.3 and Box 3.6). Such liaison helps prevent the many inappropriate acute admissions to hospital that can very seriously detract from the last few weeks of life of a patient with lung cancer.

## Further reading

NICE. Referral Guidelines for Suspected Cancer. NICE Clinical Guideline No. 27. National Institute for Health & Clinical Excellence, London 2005: http://www.nice.org.uk.

See also references to clinical guidelines for lung cancer in Table 3.1.

## CHAPTER 4

# Diagnosis and Staging

*Fergus Gleeson, Mike O'Doherty and Tom Treasure*

---

**OVERVIEW**

- Until there is a proven diagnosis all discussions with the patient are speculative; diagnosis is a critical early step in the cancer journey.
- Treatment is determined by accurate staging.
- This chapter deals with the fundamental elements of case management.
- The investigations are described in the usual sequence in which they should be performed, but not all are required in all cases.

---

Box 4.1 **The division of lung cancer types and relevant treatment**

- Small-cell lung cancers (SCLC) are nearly always disseminated when first discovered and surgery is unavailing, but they respond rapidly (if only temporarily) to chemotherapy.
- Non-small cell cancers (NSCLC) can be cured surgically if at a favourable stage.

---

In a patient with a lung lesion suspected to be cancer, the objectives of investigation are as follows:

1 To make or exclude the diagnosis as efficiently as possible. If it is not cancer an alternative diagnosis should be made if possible;

2 To determine, in the case of a diagnosis of cancer, whether it is primary or secondary. If it is primary, it should be categorised into small-cell lung cancer (SCLC; about 20% of cases) or non-small cell lung cancer (NSCLC); and

3 To define the stage of the cancer in order to plan appropriate management; metastases to nodes or other organs may preclude curative radiotherapy or surgery.

## Cancer types and their prognosis

Lung cancer is broadly divided into small-cell and non-small cell types. There are two reasons for this, as shown in Box 4.1. Overall SCLC has a worse prognosis than NSCLC, with a median life expectancy if untreated from presentation of 30 days. Life expectancy for patients with untreated stage I–III NSCLC is a median of six months. NSCLC may be further subdivided into adenocarcinoma and squamous cell carcinoma, but treatment is based upon staging and not cell type. Further distinctions into neuroendocrine and bronchoalveolar carcinomas are outside the scope of this chapter but the same diagnostic methods apply.

## Staging

SCLC is classified simply as either limited stage or extensive stage. The initial treatment for either form is chemotherapy; radiotherapy is administered to patients whose disease is limited to what can be encompassed in a radiotherapy field.

NSCLC is treated according to stage, and the results of treatment are stage dependent. Tumours are classified according to the tumour node metastasis (TNM) staging system. Clinical classification (cTNM) is determined by imaging and biopsy prior to surgery, and pathological classification (pTNM) is determined based on information from the tissues removed during surgery (Box 4.2). Both use descriptions of the local tumour (T stage), the degree of lymph node involvement (N stage) and the presence of metastases (M stage). T, N and M elements are further subclassified as stage I to IV. Each classification indicates a different life expectancy and influences treatment decisions. This staging system also enables published results of different treatment regimens to be compared (Table 4.1; see also Chapter 9, Figure 9.1). The sixth edition of the TNM classification is currently being revised.

## Imaging techniques

Different imaging and interventional techniques are available for diagnosing and staging lung cancer. The choice, sequence and relative value of these methods varies but each technique has its strengths and weaknesses, as summarised in Table 4.2.

### Chest radiograph

A clinical suspicion of lung cancer should lead to a chest X-ray (CXR; Figure 4.1), which is the most commonly performed radiographic examination worldwide. The cancer itself may be seen as a nodule in the lung field or a mass adjacent to other structures.

---

*ABC of Lung Cancer.* Edited by I. Hunt, M. Muers and T. Treasure. © 2009
Blackwell Publishing, ISBN: 978-1-4051-4652-4.

## Box 4.2 Proposed definitions for T, N and M descriptors for upcoming (2008) 7th revision of the TNM classification for lung cancer (Goldstraw et al. 2007)

### Primary tumour (T)

- **TX:** Primary tumour cannot be assessed, or tumour proven by the presence of malignant cells in sputum or bronchial washings but not visualised by imaging or bronchoscopy
- **T0:** No evidence of primary tumour
- **Tis:** Carcinoma in situ
- **T1:** Tumour <3 cm in greatest dimensions surrounded by lung or visceral pleura, without bronchoscopic evidence of invasion more proximal than the lobar bronchus. (i.e., not in the main bronchus)[a]
- **T1a:** Tumour ≤2 cm in greatest dimension
- **T1b:** Tumour >2 cm but ≤3 cm in greatest dimension
- **T2:** Tumour >3 cm but ≤7 cm or tumour with any of the following features (T2 tumours with these features are classfied T2a if ≤5 cm)
  Involves main bronchus, ≥2 cm distal to the carina
  Invades the visceral pleura
  Associated with atelectasis or obstructive pneumonitis that extends to the hilar region but does not involve the entire lung
- **T2a:** Tumour >3 cm but ≤5 cm in greatest dimension
- **T2b:** Tumour >5 cm but ≤7 cm in greatest dimension
- **T3:** Tumour >7 cm or one that directly invades any of the following: chest wall (including superior sulcus tumours), diaphragm, phrenic nerve, mediastinal pleura, parietal pericardium; or tumour in the main bronchus <2 cm distal to the carina[a] but without involvement of the carina; or associated atelectasis or obstructive pneumonitis of the entire lung or separate tumour nodule (s) in the same lobe
- **T4:** Tumour of any size that invades any of the following: mediastinum, heart, great vessels, trachea, recurrent laryngeal nerve, esophagus, vertebral body, carina; separate tumour nodules (s) in a different ipsilateral lobe

### Regional lymph nodes (N)

- **NX:** Regional lymph nodes cannot be assessed
- **N0:** No regional lymph node metastasis
- **N1:** Metastasis in ipsilateral peribronchial and/or ipsilateral hilar lymph nodes and intrapulmonary nodes, including involvement by direct extension
- **N2:** Metastasis in ipsilateral mediastinal and/or subcarinal lymph node (s).
- **N3:** Metastasis in contralateral mediastinal, contralateral hilar, ipsilateral or contralateral scalene, or supraclavicular lymph node (s).

### Distant metastasis (N)

- **MX:** Distant metastasis cannot be assessed
- **M0:** No distant metastasis
- **M1:** Distant metastasis
- **M1a:** Separate tumour nodules (s) in a contralateral lobe; tumour with pleural nodules or malignant pleural (or pericardial) effusion[b]
- **M1b:** Distant metastasis

[a]The uncommon superficial spreading tumour of any size with its invasive component limited to the bronchial wall, which may extend proximally to the main bronchus is also classified as T1.

[b]Most pleural (and pericardial) effusions with lung cancer are due to tumour. In a few patients, however multiple cytopathologic examinations of pleural (pericardial) fluid are negative for tumour, and the fluid is nonbloody and is not an exudate. Where these elements and clinical judgment dictate that the effusion is not related to the tumour, the effusion should be excluded as a staging element and the patient should be classified as T1, T2, T3, or T4.

**Table 4.1** Stage definitions and five-year survival figures for non-small cell lung cancer (NSCLC) based on current (6th) TNM classification (see also Figure 9.1).

| Stage | Definition | Clinical staging | Pathological staging |
|---|---|---|---|
| IA | T1 N1 M0 | 61% | 67% |
| IB | T2 N0 M0 | 38% | 57% |
| IIA | T1 N1 M0 | 34% | 55% |
| IIB | T2 N1 M0<br>T3 N0 M0 | 22–34% | 38–55% |
| IIIA | T3 N1 M0<br>T1 N2 M0<br>T2 N2 M0<br>T3 N2 M0 | 9–13% | 23–25% |
| IIIB | T4 N0 M0<br>T4 N1 M0<br>T4 N2 M0<br>T1 N3 M0<br>T2 N3 M0<br>T3 N3 M0<br>T4 N3 M0 | 1–8% | – |
| IV | Any T, any N, M1 | 1% | – |

**Table 4.2** Methods of investigation and their relative value or usefulness in making a pathological diagnosis and for staging.

| | Pathological* diagnosis | T stage | N stage | M stage |
|---|---|---|---|---|
| CXR | – | + | + | Chance observations** |
| CT | – | +++ | ++ | ++ |
| CT-guided biopsy | +++ | – | + | +++ |
| Bronchoscopy | +++ | + | ++ | – |
| PET-CT | + | +++ | +++ | +++ |
| Mediastinoscopy | ++ | + | +++ | – |
| Ultrasound | + | + | + | + |
| Ultrasound biopsy | +++ | + | + | +++ |
| MRI | | +++ | ++ | ++ |

*In the clinical context the information on imaging alone may make pursuit of tissue diagnosis unnecessary and inappropriate, but the standard of care is to prove the diagnosis under the microscope; ** For example, bone metastases in the clavicle or pathological fractures of ribs; –, not generally useful; +, limited use; ++, often useful; +++, usually useful; CT, computed tomography; CXR, chest X-ray; MRI, magnetic resonance imaging; PET, positron emission tomography.

Alternatively, its presence may be evident in the form of lymph node enlargement, pleural effusion, lung collapse or consolidation, or a combination of these abnormalities (Figure 4.2). A small percentage of cancers will either not be apparent on the initial CXR or missed in reporting. If suspicion remains then further investigation, usually a computed tomography (CT) scan, should be performed.

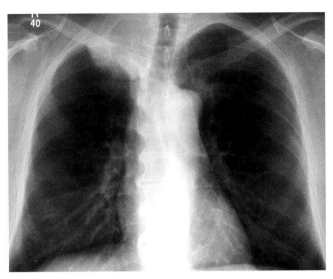

**Figure 4.1** A right apical tumour seen on a chest X-ray (CXR) in a patient presenting with a cough and right shoulder pain.

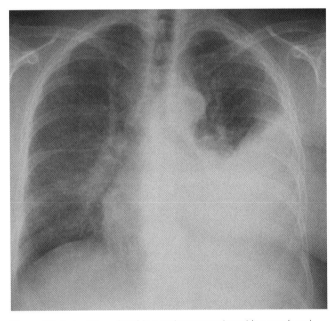

**Figure 4.2** A chest X-ray (CXR) in a patient presenting with a cough and weight loss, showing a large left-sided pleural effusion, preventing the underlying carcinoma from being visualised.

## Computed tomography

The next usual investigation is a contrast-enhanced CT scan. Multislice scanners image the chest and liver in less than 10 seconds. CT appearance determines whether CT-guided biopsy, bronchoscopy or surgery is used to make a tissue diagnosis. The radiologist may support a diagnosis of malignancy from evidence of invasion of the chest wall or mediastinum, or may suspect metastases to lymph nodes or other organs (Figures 4.3 and 4.4); however, a diagnosis of cancer relies on examination of the tissue by a pathologist. The main role of CT is in the staging of confirmed cancer (Figure 4.5). In the presence of lung cancer, lymph nodes with a short axis diameter of 1 cm or more are specific for metastases in two-thirds of cases.

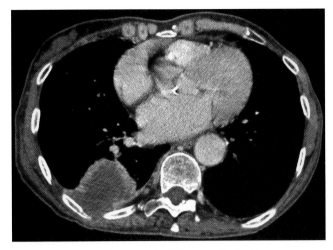

**Figure 4.3** A computed tomography (CT) scan confirming that a mass seen on chest X-ray (CXR) is malignant by showing chest wall invasion posteriorly.

## Computed tomography-guided needle biopsy

In expertly selected cases a tissue diagnosis can be made in up to 90% of biopsies, including small lesions (Figure 4.6).

## Bronchoscopy

Fibreoptic bronchoscopy is performed routinely at very low risk in outpatients (Figure 4.7). It is the technique of choice to obtain tissue for diagnosis from tumours seen lying centrally on CT or from those associated with a collapsed lung (Figure 4.8). Transbronchial needle aspiration biopsy (TBNA) is an increasingly common technique when making a tissue diagnosis of both the primary cancer and lymph nodes adjacent to the airways. Endobronchial ultrasound (EBUS) is likely to have a significant impact in helping to diagnose and stage patients with suspected lung cancer.

## The goal of curative or palliative treatment

At this point in the investigative pathway the diagnosis of cancer and the stage of the primary tumour (T stage) are usually known. If there is good evidence that there is lymph node (N stage) involvement or distant metastases (M stage), then the cancer is not curable by local measures (surgery or radiotherapy) and further investigations are not usually required to make a treatment plan. If it is proposed to treat by surgery, radiotherapy with the possibility of cure, or combination therapy then more detailed staging is required.

## Positron emission tomography

Positron emission tomography (PET) scanning relies on increased metabolism of glucose by the cancer as the means of detection (see Chapter 3, Box 3.3). Deoxyglucose labelled with radioactive 18-fluorine ($^{18}$F-fluorodeoxygluose or FDG) is injected intravenously. Glucose (including FDG) is readily taken up by malignant cells but deoxyglucose cannot be metabolised completely in the normal glucose metabolic pathway and thus becomes trapped and accumulates as $^{18}$FDG-6-phosphate (Figure 4.9). CT combined with

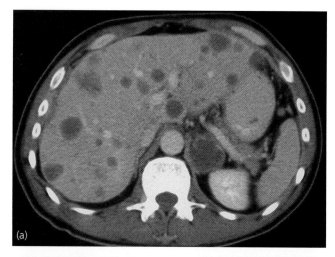

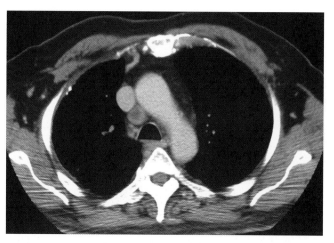

**Figure 4.5** A mass seen on a computed tomography (CT) scan is associated with a right paratracheal node. Mediastinoscopy would be required to confirm that the node was enlarged secondary to metastatic involvement.

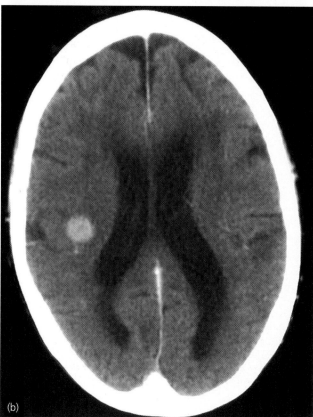

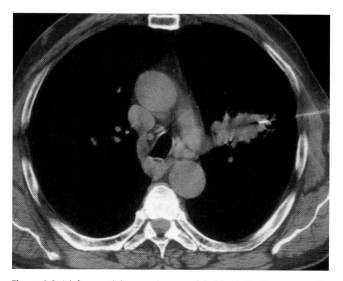

**Figure 4.6** A left upper lobe mass is successfully biopsied using computed tomography (CT) image guidance.

**Figure 4.4** (a) and (b) Multiple liver metastases and a cerebral metastasis seen on a computed tomography (CT) scan in a patient with a mass seen on chest X-ray (CXR) and CT. The presence of the metastases allows a CT diagnosis of malignancy, but a tissue diagnosis is still required to allow differentiation of small-cell (as in this case) from non-small cell lung cancer, and to plan treatment.

PET (PET-CT) enables the anatomical location of lesions containing the FDG derivative.

PET is a very sensitive method for the evaluation of lymphade-nopathy, so no further investigation is required if lymph nodes detected during CT staging appear negative by PET. The specificity of PET-CT for nodal involvement is 85%; hence, it may be deemed necessary to obtain tissue confirmation if the PET result is all that stands in the way of an attempt at surgical cure (see the section on mediastinoscopy). PET-CT is also being evaluated in radiotherapy planning and may be helpful in patients with pulmonary collapse and/or consolidation, since the FDG uptake may separate the tumour from the consolidated lung.

The most important use of PET-CT in the evaluation of patients for potential curative treatment is in the detection of remote metastases (Figure 4.10). Almost 20% of patients have metastases that were not detected by staging CT scans. These patients are spared unavailing surgery for lung cancer.

Confirmation of the presence of metastatic disease detected during the initial staging CT scan or subsequent PET-CT scans is most commonly achieved by image-guided biopsy. When possible this method should be used for providing a tissue diagnosis because confirmation of distant metastases (M1) allows immediate classification as a stage IV disease.

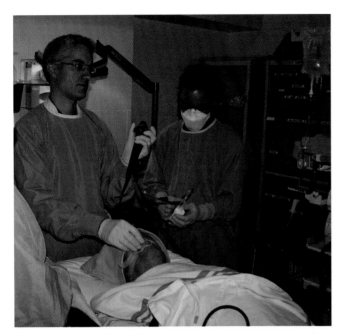

**Figure 4.7** Flexible bronchoscopy is performed under sedation in the endoscopy suite via the nasal or oral route.

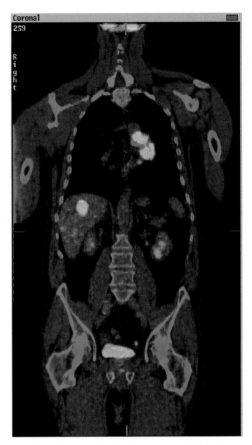

**Figure 4.9** A combined positron emission tomography and computed tomography (PET-CT) scan showing a large left upper lobe mass with a necrotic centre. Note the increased isotope activity in the rim of the tumour with no activity in the necrotic centre.

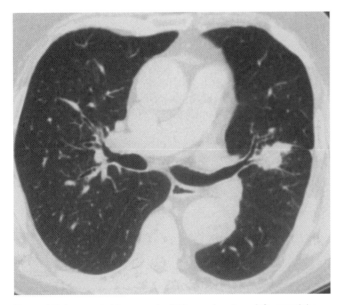

**Figure 4.8** A computed tomography (CT) scan showing a left upper lobe lesion with a bronchus passing directly into it. This suggested, correctly, that bronchoscopy would be positive.

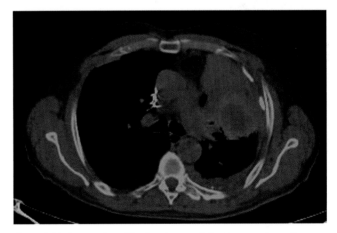

**Figure 4.10** A coronal combined positron emission tomography and computed tomography (PET-CT) scan showing a left upper lobe/hilar tumour and also a liver metastasis demonstrating increased isotope activity. The liver lesion was barely visible on the CT scan performed prior to the PET scan.

## Mediastinoscopy and other surgical staging methods

Confirmation of mediastinal nodal involvement is necessary in NSCLC if there is no evidence of metastatic disease elsewhere. CT is a sensitive method of detecting nodal enlargement, but is not specific for malignant involvement. It is now possible to biopsy enlarged mediastinal nodes at bronchoscopy, but surgical staging using mediastinoscopy or anterior mediastinotomy may be necessary.

Spread to mediastinal lymph nodes is an important watershed between inoperable lung cancer and cases where surgery should be offered. These nodes sit amongst the large mediastinal vessels and can be sampled surgically but not by needle biopsy. The patient must be admitted to a thoracic surgical unit for this procedure.

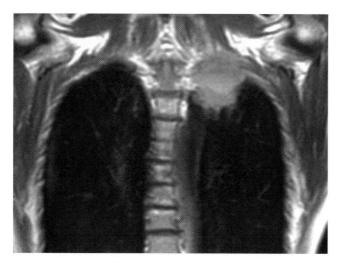

**Figure 4.11** A coronal T1 weighted magnetic resonance imaging (MRI) scan showing invasion of the left apical pleura and involvement of the brachial plexus by an apical carcinoma.

Under general anaesthetic an instrument is introduced in the pretracheal tissue plane and can be advanced as far as the carina. In expert hands the risk of serious bleeding is in the order of 1 in 500, but if it occurs it can be catastrophic.

## Ultrasound

Ultrasound (US) has a limited but highly useful role in the diagnosis of lung cancer. It may be used to confirm fixity of pulmonary lesions to the chest wall, if there is doubt on CT, or to help to characterise liver lesions seen on staging CT scans. However, it is most frequently used to guide interventional procedures such as pleural aspiration, biopsy of pulmonary masses abutting the chest wall, biopsy of liver or rib metastases, or more recently to guide biopsy of supraclavicular lymph nodes. US-guided intervention is safer, quicker and cheaper than other interventional techniques.

## Magnetic resonance imaging

CT and magnetic resonance imaging (MRI) can be used interchangeably in staging, with both providing high quality anatomical information. The special place of MRI as opposed to CT is in the accurate assessment of apical tumours, which provide evidence of adjacent soft tissue invasion, in particular of the brachial plexus (Figure 4.11). Occasionally MRI may be used to characterise liver or adrenal lesions seen on staging CT scans.

Most patients with lung cancer should be imaged and investigated using standard techniques and diagnostic pathways. It is important that a tissue diagnosis is obtained and the patient correctly staged. Once these steps have been achieved then a treatment plan can be devised. This may involve an attempted cure with either surgery or radical radiotherapy in patients with stages I to IIIA; alternatively, palliative therapy would be offered to patients with an impairment of lung function that renders them unsuitable for radical treatment, or for patients with advanced disease (i.e. stages IIIB and IV; Table 4.1). PET-CT is currently reserved for those patients that are considered operable or are being considered for radical radiotherapy.

## Further reading

Alberts WM & Collice GM, eds. Diagnosis and management of lung cancer: ACCP evidence-based guidelines. *Chest* 2003; **123(Suppl 1):** 1S–337S.

Goldstraw P, Crowley J, Chansky K *et al.* The IASLC Lung Cancer Staging Project: proposals for the revision of the TNM stage groupings in the forthcoming (seventh) edition of the TNM classification of malignant Tumours. *Journal of Thoracic Oncology* 2007; **2(8):** 706–714.

Lababede O, Meziane MA & Rice TW. TNM staging of lung cancer: a quick reference chart. *Chest* 1999; **115:** 233–235.

NICE. *Referral Guidelines for Suspected Cancer.* NICE Clinical Guideline No. 27. National Institute for Health & Clinical Excellence, London 2005: http://www.nice.org.uk

# CHAPTER 5

# Small-Cell Lung Cancer

*Penella Woll, Patricia Hunt and Michael Snee*

---

**OVERVIEW**

- Small-cell lung cancer (SCLC) has a clinical course and response to treatment that is sufficiently distinct from other lung cancers as to merit separate consideration.
- SCLC metastasises early and is a systemic disease at presentation in nearly all cases; surgery and radiotherapy are not used in isolation.
- Rather than using the tumour node metastasis (TNM) classification system, SCLC is staged simply into either limited or extensive disease.
- Combined chemotherapy and radiotherapy is the treatment of choice.

---

**Table 5.1** Paraneoplastic syndromes associated with small-cell lung cancer (SCLC).

| Secreted peptide or hormone | Mechanism | Clinical presentation |
|---|---|---|
| Vasopressin (antidiuretic hormone, ADH) | Low serum sodium | Weakness, blackouts |
| Adrenocorticotrophin (ACTH) | High cortisol | Cushing's syndrome |
| Atrial natriuretic peptide (ANP) | Low serum sodium | Weakness, blackouts |
| Granulocyte colony stimulating factor (G-CSF) | High WBC | Asymptomatic |
| Paraneoplastic encephalomyelitis/sensory neuropathy (PEM/SN) | Anti-Hu antibodies | Sensory neuropathy, cerebellar ataxia, pseudo-obstruction |
| Lambert Eaton myasthenic syndrome (LEMS) | Voltage-gated calcium channel antibodies | Proximal muscle weakness, autonomic symptoms |

Small-cell lung cancer (SCLC) comprises 15–20% of all lung cancers. Its pathological characteristics, clinical course and response to treatment distinguish it from other 'non-small cell' lung cancers. Indeed, it was the observation that SCLC patients fared so poorly after surgery but did respond to chemotherapy that led to the distinction between SCLC and all other lung cancers.

Under the microscope, SCLC cells appear closely packed together, with large nuclei and scanty cytoplasm, leading to the descriptive name of 'oat cell' carcinoma. SCLC grows rapidly without laying down a supportive stroma, so the tumours are friable and characteristically fragment when biopsied. The tumours have the capacity to synthesise a wide variety of hormones and peptides, which can cause puzzling clinical presentations (Table 5.1).

## Classification and investigations

SCLC metastasises early, so it is treated as a systemic disease from the time of diagnosis. After the pathological diagnosis has been established, and based on clinical examination and a computed tomography (CT) scan of the thorax and liver, patients are classified simply as having limited or extensive-stage disease (Box 5.1). This clearly separates the better from the worse prognosis patients and is useful when discussing the treatment options. Radiotherapists use a more pragmatic definition of limited disease; i.e. that which can

---

**Box 5.1 Staging classification for small-cell lung cancer (SCLC)**

- **Limited stage:** disease confined to one hemithorax, including hilar and mediastinal lymph nodes, ipsilateral and contralateral supra-clavicular fossa lymph nodes, and ipsilateral pleural effusion.
- **Extensive stage:** disease without the above.

---

be encompassed by a 12 × 15 cm field of radiation. More detailed staging classifications are unnecessary.

Additional investigations (such as bone or brain scans) are carried out when clinically indicated (for example, if the patient has bony pain or headaches), but they are not routinely performed. In addition to extensive stage, several other adverse prognostic features have been identified (Box 5.2). These include poor performance status (PS) and raised serum lactate dehydrogenase (LDH). It should be noted that age does not consistently influence prognosis. Many clinicians use a scoring system to identify patients with a better prognosis, for whom the chance of longer survival merits

*ABC of Lung Cancer*. Edited by I. Hunt, M. Muers and T. Treasure. © 2009 Blackwell Publishing, ISBN: 978-1-4051-4652-4.

Box 5.2 **Adverse prognostic factors for patients with small-cell lung cancer (SCLC), in order of decreasing importance**

- World Health Organisation (WHO) performance status >2
- Raised serum lactate dehydrogenase (LDH)
- Extensive stage disease
- Male sex
- Multiple metastatic sites
- Low serum sodium

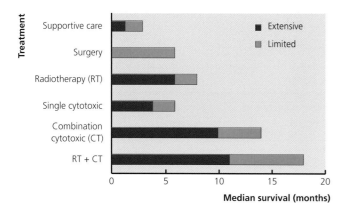

**Figure 5.1** The impact of small-cell lung cancer (SCLC) treatment on survival.

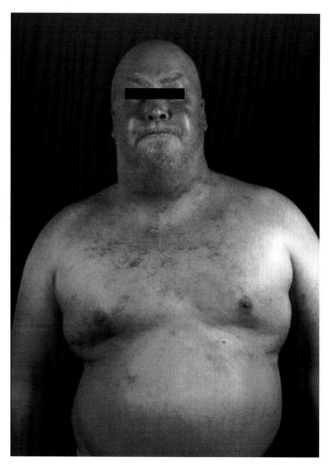

**Figure 5.2** Superior vena caval obstruction due to small-cell lung cancer (SCLC).

more intensive treatment, and those with a worse prognosis, for whom symptom control with minimal toxicity is the aim.

## Prognosis and treatment

Without treatment, the median survival is six weeks for patients with extensive disease and 12 weeks for those with limited disease (Figure 5.1). Because SCLC is considered a systemic disease in the majority of patients, systemic chemotherapy is the treatment of choice. In many cases this is given in conjunction with radiotherapy. Where surgery is performed (usually because it was not possible to obtain a pathological diagnosis prior to operation), adjuvant chemotherapy is recommended. Radiotherapy is no longer used in isolation. Since the introduction of chemotherapy treatment for SCLC in the 1970s, patient survival has improved considerably. However, despite this the majority of patients still die from their cancer.

## Chemotherapy treatment

SCLC is extremely sensitive to chemotherapy, with more than 80% of patients achieving substantial disease shrinkage. Because these tumours have little stroma, the response to chemotherapy can be extremely rapid. For this reason, chemotherapy remains the preferred treatment modality even when there are critical symptoms from the local disease, such as superior vena caval obstruction (Figure 5.2; see Chapter 11, Figure 11.2). Patients typically experience significant relief of symptoms within 24–48 hours of receiving chemotherapy (Figure 5.3). Because there is a high chance of

symptomatic benefit and prolongation of life, chemotherapy is even offered to patients with very advanced disease, although the risks and benefits have to be carefully explained to such patients and their families.

There is good evidence that combining several chemotherapy drugs gives better symptom relief, disease control and survival than single-agent chemotherapy (Figure 5.1). Typically, chemotherapy is given using injectable and oral agents at 3–4 week intervals, up to a maximum of six cycles. There is no evidence that longer courses or 'maintenance' chemotherapy are beneficial. Chemotherapy can be given in the inpatient and day care setting in both cancer units and cancer centres (Figure 5.4).

On the day of chemotherapy administration, patients are assessed by the medical team and specialist nurses to ensure that the adverse effects of the previous cycle have resolved and to assess the effectiveness of the treatment. Specialist chemotherapy nurses also ensure the safe administration of the drugs, and this provides a good opportunity for the nurses to address patients' needs and to ensure that they are fully supported within the community.

Active chemotherapy drugs include platinums (cisplatin, carboplatin), anthracyclines (doxorubicin, epirubicin), alkylating agents (cyclophosphamide, ifosfamide) and mitotic inhibitors (vinca alkaloids, taxanes, etoposide). Combinations are chosen to have additive efficacy but different toxicities, such as cisplatin

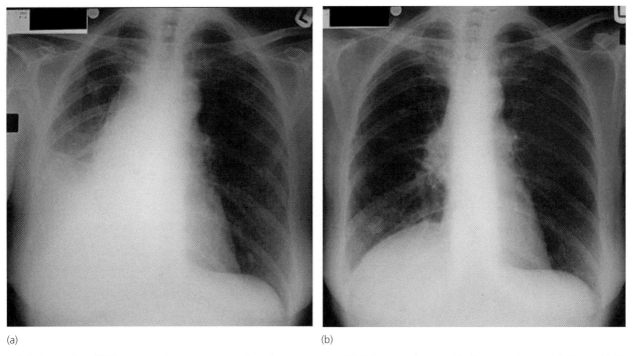

(a)                                                                                                    (b)

**Figure 5.3** A chest X-ray (CXR) demonstrating the response of small-cell lung cancer (SCLC) to one cycle of combination chemotherapy. (a) 15 May. (b) 9 June.

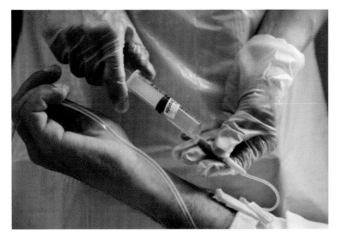

**Figure 5.4** A patient receiving chemotherapy for small-cell lung cancer (SCLC).

and etoposide or cyclophosphamide, doxorubicin and vincristine. Recent evidence suggests that platinum-containing regimens should be preferred, as they are associated with better survival and less mouth ulceration (mucositis) and bone marrow suppression, resulting in a lower risk of life-threatening infections.

## Combination chemoradiotherapy

In patients with limited-stage SCLC, combination treatment with systemic chemotherapy and radiotherapy to the chest leads to significantly better survival than either treatment alone. The median survival rate for patients with limited disease is 18 months and up to 10% of patients are alive at five years. Radiotherapy can either be given concurrently (early) with chemotherapy or after completing it (late).

The brain is a common site for secondary spread (metastases) from SCLC, even in patients who have had a good response to chemotherapy. This is because the brain is relatively protected from chemotherapy by the blood-brain barrier. Prophylactic cranial irradiation (PCI) has been proposed as a means to prevent brain metastases in patients whose primary disease has responded well to chemotherapy. Recent clinical trials have shown that PCI is effective in patients with both limited and extensive-stage SCLC. It substantially reduces the risk of developing brain metastases (by about 50%) and leads to a smaller but significant improvement in survival.

## Adverse effects of treatment

The most feared adverse effects of chemotherapy are sickness and hair loss. In actuality, all of the adverse effects are manageable in the vast majority of patients. Nausea can usually be well controlled with 5-hydroxytryptamine 3 (5HT3) antagonists such as granisetron, steroids and domperidone or metoclopramide. Vomiting is now unusual. Although hair loss is unavoidable with the majority of chemotherapy regimens, it lasts for the duration of treatment and then the hair regrows. However, the hair may not grow back fully following cranial radiotherapy. The most serious adverse effect of chemotherapy is immunosuppression due to bone marrow suppression, which is at its worst 9–12 days following treatment. Patients with abnormally low levels of circulating neutrophils (i.e. that are neutropenic) can rapidly succumb to life-threatening infections at this time, and must be

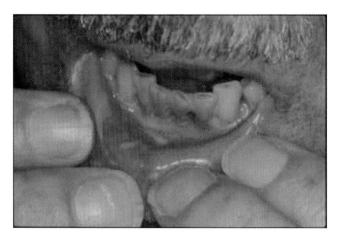

**Figure 5.5** Mouth ulceration due to cytotoxic chemotherapy.

counselled about the importance of discussing any new symptoms or fevers with their hospital team. As many lung cancer patients have bronchial obstruction at presentation, there is a high risk of chest infections following the first chemotherapy treatment, which is halved in subsequent cycles. Many centres recommend prophylactic antibiotics during the first chemotherapy cycle for this reason. Additional adverse effects include tiredness, soreness of the mouth (mucositis; Figure 5.5) and damage to peripheral nerves (neuropathy), which may necessitate dose modifications. Following thoracic radiotherapy many patients experience unpleasant oesophagitis (Figure 5.6), which requires treatment with sucralfate and opiate analgesia along with dietary advice. Radiation-induced inflammation of the spinal cord (myelitis) is a rare but serious adverse effect.

## Follow-up

After completing chemoradiotherapy for SCLC, patients should return to near-normal levels of activity, with no residual symptoms and very little residual toxicity. However, this may take time and may require ongoing support from the community and hospital teams. Patients can be followed up by an oncologist, chest physician or lung cancer specialist nurse, who will typically review the patient at bimonthly intervals. Regular X-rays and scans are not required. Unfortunately, many of the patients will relapse within two years of diagnosis. Second-line chemotherapy can be offered, but thoracic and cranial radiotherapy cannot be repeated. The response rate to second-line chemotherapy is lower than first-line treatment (30 *vs.* 80%) and the duration of the response is likely to be shorter. Nevertheless, most patients have had a good experience of first-line treatment, often with dramatic symptom improvement, and are keen to repeat the experience. Treatment can be given with the same chemotherapy regimen if the benefits lasted for more than

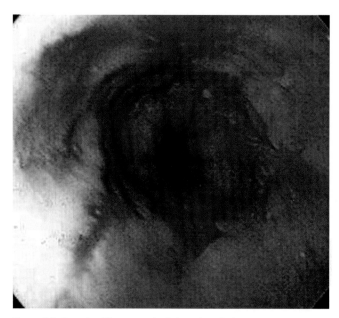

**Figure 5.6** Oesophagitis as a result of thoracic radiotherapy.

six months. More commonly, alternative chemotherapy drugs are used in the hope of overcoming drug resistance. Palliative radiotherapy can be offered for localised symptoms, such as bony pain. A wide range of palliative approaches (such as opiates) and procedures (for example superior vena caval stenting) are available (see Chapter 11), but for many patients second-line chemotherapy offers the best chance of controlling their symptoms.

## Further reading

Auperin A, Arriagada R, Pignon JP, *et al.* Prophylactic cranial irradiation for patients with small-cell lung cancer in complete remission. Prophylactic Cranial Irradiation Overview Collaborative Group. *New England Journal of Medicine* 1999; **341**(7): 476–484.

Girling DJ. Comparison of oral etoposide and standard intravenous multidrug chemotherapy for small-cell lung cancer: a stopped multicentre randomised trial. Medical Research Council Lung Cancer Working Party. *Lancet* 1996; **348**(9027): 563–566.

Pignon JP, Arriagada R, Ihde DC. A meta-analysis of thoracic radiotherapy for small-cell lung cancer. *New England Journal of Medicine* 1992; **327**: 1618–1624.

Slotman B, Faivre-Finn C, Kramer G, *et al.* for the EORTC Radiation Oncology Group and Lung Cancer Group. Prophylactic cranial irradiation in extensive small-cell lung cancer. *New England Journal of Medicine* 2007; **357**: 664–672.

Sundstrom S, Bremnes RM, Kaasa S, *et al.* Cisplatin and etoposide regimen is superior to cyclophosphamide, epirubicin, and vincristine regimen in small-cell lung cancer: results from a randomized phase III trial with 5 years' follow-up. *Journal of Clinical Oncology* 2002; **20**(24): 4665–4672.

# CHAPTER 6

# Malignant Pleural Mesothelioma

*Carol Tan, Fergus Gleeson and Tom Treasure*

**OVERVIEW**

- Mesothelioma is an aggressive tumour with a poor prognosis that is associated with previous asbestos exposure.
- It is no longer considered to be rare and an epidemic in Europe is expected over the next 20 years.
- Early referral to a multidisciplinary cancer team with experience of mesothelioma care should be considered on suspicion.
- Response to most available therapies is currently still poor and treatment should ideally be considered within clinical trials, where possible.

## Epidemiological trends

Malignant pleural mesothelioma is a cancer attributable in nearly all cases to asbestos exposure, typically 30–40 years before disease onset (Figure 6.1). Europe is facing an epidemic of the disease following the widespread use of asbestos from the 1950s up until about 1980 (Figure 6.2). The death rate from mesothelioma in Europe is predicted to peak between 2010 and 2015. In the USA the incidence of mesothelioma has plateaued and may actually be declining because asbestos use was controlled earlier. In the UK, where there is still a perception that this is a rare cancer, it kills more people a year than either melanoma or cancer of the cervix, which are both widely publicised and very familiar to the public at large. There were 153 registered deaths from the disease in 1968, rising to 1862 in 2002, and there are likely be 60,000 deaths over the next 45 years. Following this peak, the number of deaths is expected to decline, reflecting the subsequent control of asbestos in the 1980s. It is prevalent in Australia and unrestricted asbestos use in many Third World countries will provide a large number of cases in the life times of the present working generation.

It is an extraordinary situation and may be unique, in that we can predict the number of cases but can do nothing to prevent them. While we can at least be confident that the current epidemic will peak and

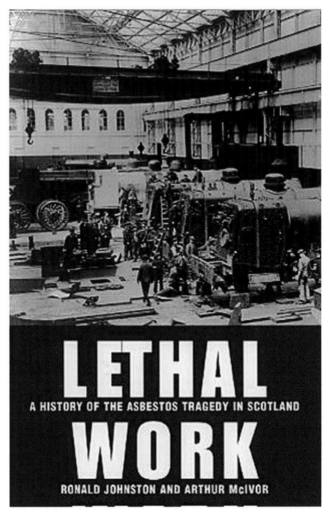

**Figure 6.1** The cover of a book recently published on the history of asbestos use in Glasgow, Scotland.

subsequently decline in the coming decades in Britain, there is no such reassurance in the developing world.

## The history of asbestos use

Asbestos was highly valued as an insulator and fire retardant and was widely used in construction, ship-building and the manufacture

*ABC of Lung Cancer*. Edited by I. Hunt, M. Muers and T. Treasure. © 2009 Blackwell Publishing, ISBN: 978-1-4051-4652-4.

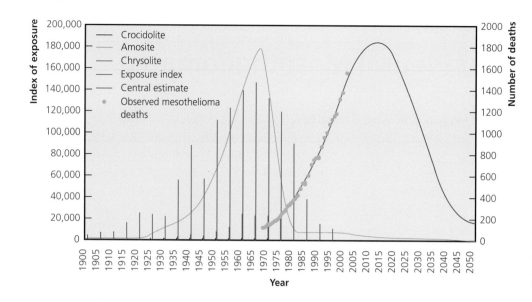

**Figure 6.2** An illustration of the likely course of mesothelioma-related deaths in the UK among males aged 20–89 years, compared to the estimated/projected exposure index for different types of asbestos.

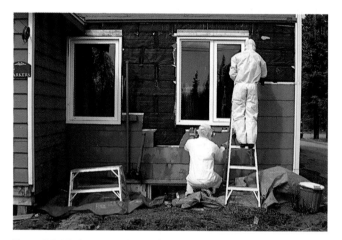

**Figure 6.3** Modern precautions utilised when removing asbestos during the refurbishment of asbestos-laden buildings.

of household appliances. This led to a wide distribution of asbestos in the environment. Although those that were industrially exposed face the highest risk per thousand workers, the millions more that were casually exposed such as carpenters, painters and decorators, heating engineers, garage mechanics, do-it-yourself home improvement enthusiasts, and the families of workers who brought asbestos dust home on their clothes, present the higher number of cases. If current control measures are not adhered to, asbestos removal workers are now potentially at the highest risk, as are workers involved in the refurbishment, repair or maintenance of buildings (Figure 6.3).

## Presenting features

Mesothelioma is a slow-growing primary cancer originating in the parietal pleura, thickening it irregularly with a pebbled appearance. Over time, the cancer grows relentlessly into adjacent structures including the chest wall, visceral pleura, lung, diaphragm, pericardiu and the heart. The commonest

presentations are cough and breathlessness due to pleural effusion, and pain due to tumour growth into the chest wall. These symptoms can be mistaken for a chest infection and occasionally several courses of antibiotics may be prescribed before a more sinister underlying diagnosis is suspected. Other non-specific symptoms include anorexia, weight loss, weakness and fever.

Pleural mesothelioma is almost always unilateral and if there is an effusion, clinical examination reveals a dull percussion note and reduced or absent breath sounds associated with reduced chest expansion on the affected side. Patients with locally advanced disease may have a palpable chest wall mass. This may also happen after previous investigation by needle aspiration or biopsy as this cancer has a strong predilection for growing along a needle track. Any of these features may prompt a chest X-ray (CXR; Figure 6.4).

## Confirming the diagnosis

Clinically it cannot be distinguished from any other cause of malignant effusion. A strong history of asbestos exposure raises suspicion, but asbestos was so widespread that the absence of a clear history of exposure is almost valueless in excluding the diagnosis. Prompt referral to a chest clinic at this point is usually the best course of action.

The radiological appearances may be highly suggestive of mesothelioma, but pathological proof is essential in nearly all cases. Without it we cannot open a sensible discussion with the patient or embark on a management plan. There are also issues of compensation and litigation that cannot be pursued without proof. If pleural fluid can be aspirated for diagnosis and/or symptom relief then a portion should be sent for cytology. This may be diagnostic in a minority of cases (about 1 in 4); however, no reliance should be placed on a negative result.

A computed tomography (CT) scan is usually the best next step in advancing the diagnosis, commonly revealing nodular pleural thickening underlying the pleural effusion. In more advanced disease there is contraction of the hemithorax as the

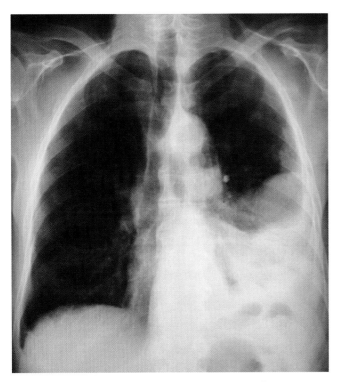

**Figure 6.4** A chest X-ray (CXR) demonstrating left pleural effusion.

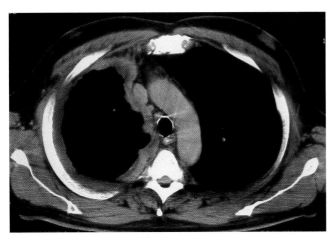

**Figure 6.5** A computed tomography (CT) scan showing a constricting pleural tumour surrounding the right lung and contacting the right hemithorax.

tumour wraps around the lung, thus restricting full expansion (Figure 6.5). It is often possible to biopsy the pleural thickening under CT guidance, and this provides the diagnosis in 80–90% of patients. Alternatively, or if this fails, surgical biopsy is needed. This is usually obtained as part of video-assisted thorascopic surgery (VATS), which is commonly performed in a thoracic unit but may be carried out by chest physicians under local anaesthesia and sedation in some units.

A word of caution: the time can pass by even with the best care. Until a CXR is performed, the focus will not move to a pleural cause for breathlessness, and until the tissue diagnosis is made, appropriate treatment cannot start. Negative pleural

aspirations and repeat CXR do not advance the process. Even when histological specimens are taken the diagnosis can be difficult to confirm. Early referral to the local lung multidisciplinary cancer team is important on suspicion and they may refer on to a regional unit with more experience of mesothelioma care; they will then advise on the best route to diagnosis.

A special note: this cancer has a propensity for growing down needle aspiration and chest drain tracts to produce painful nodules, as noted above. Local radiotherapy to these sites is effective in reducing this problem and should be offered following any attempted biopsy.

## Management strategy

The management strategy is often dependent on location and stage of the cancer, as well as the performance status and symptoms of the patient. With a median survival usually cited as 6 to 12 months from time of diagnosis, treatments need to be not only effective, but given expeditiously and efficiently. Recent reports include longer survival times, but with greater awareness and better diagnostic strategies the diagnosis is being made earlier, which introduces a lead time bias in the date. Despite recent advances including more accurate staging, improvement in surgical techniques and novel chemotherapy and radiotherapy techniques, not much impact is being made on survival time; a 'cure' in mesothelioma, if ever achieved, must be very rare. A more modest but realistic objective is to get the best symptom relief we can, for the longest possible time

## The role of supportive and palliative care

In most cases the diagnosis is made when the disease is already in advanced stages. It often progresses quickly with unremitting pain and deterioration in pulmonary function and cachexia. Palliative treatment for pain, breathlessness and other symptoms may therefore be required from the outset.

## Management of breathlessness

Breathlessness may be caused by the thick cortex of tumour surrounding the lung or by a moderate to large pleural effusion. If there is pleural fluid and its aspiration or drainage relieves breathlessness, then this benefit can often be sustained by pleurodesis. This can be achieved either by VATS with talc insufflation at the time of pleural biopsy (Figure 6.6), or at the bedside by instilling talc slurry through a chest drain. Attention to technique is important if good relief is to be achieved and infection (a miserable complication) is to be avoided. Talc pleurodesis is best done early and by expert and experienced hands.

## The role of chemotherapy

Many clinical studies have assessed the role of chemotherapy for malignant mesothelioma. There is response to chemotherapy in some cases and the best choice of agents and regimens is the subject of trials. Pemetrexed has shown the best benefit in a randomised controlled trial (RCT) at the time of writing. However, the survival gains are modest and whilst there are ongoing clinical trials,

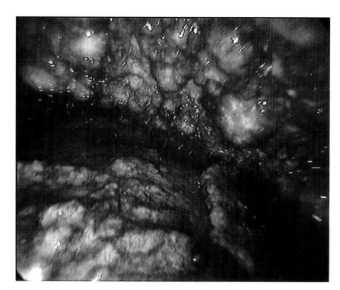

**Figure 6.6** A video-assisted thorascopic surgery (VATS) image of mesothelioma.

patients with mesothelioma should be encouraged to participate in these. As well as assessing survival gains it is important to assess benefit in terms of quality of life.

## The role of surgery

As discussed previously, surgery has important diagnostic and palliative objectives in mesothelioma. The place of surgical resection, whether in debulking of disease by one version or another of pleurectomy/decortication (P/D) or extrapleural pneumonectomy (EPP), is less clear (see Box 6.1). Mesothelioma is difficult to eradicate by virtue of its nature, extent, pattern of growth and proximity to major organs.

Although mortality and morbidity associated with more radical EPP are significant, a retrospective analysis has claimed that there is a survival advantage in select patients with early-stage disease. The best results appear to be achieved when EPP is performed with adjuvant chemotherapy and/or post operative hemithorax radiotherapy. The role of this trimodality therapy is currently being assessed within the context of a RCT (Mesothelioma and Radical Surgery, or MARS trial) in the UK; that of debulking by minimal access surgery in being investigated in the MesoVATS trial.

---

Box 6.1 **The surgical options in managing mesothelioma**

- **Pleurectomy/decortication:** removes the bulk of the tumour to allow the underlying lung to re-expand. However, complete clearance of disease is difficult and air leaks from raw lung surface are common postoperatively.
- **Extrapleural pneumonectomy (EPP):** involves *en bloc* removal of the lung within the stripped parietal pleura, together with the pericardium and diaphragm.

## The place of screening

With the impending epidemic and the thus far poor results of available treatment, the question of screening has arisen. Up until recently no reliable tumour marker for mesothelioma has been identified. However, there is now a serum marker – mesothelin, which has been shown to be highly specific and moderately sensitive for mesothelioma. The expression of this marker rises in proportion to the bulk of the disease and therefore is more likely to pick up unsuspected but already advanced disease rather than detecting early disease. Nonetheless, a negative test does not provide assurance that mesothelioma will not present in years to come. Until there are treatment options that will make a difference, it does not appear to be in the patients' best interests to go looking for disease.

## Further reading

Hodgson JT, McElvenny DM, Darnton AJ, Price MJ & Peto J. The expected burden of mesothelioma mortality in Great Britain from 2002 to 2050. *British Journal of Cancer* 2005; **92**(3): 587–593.

Johnson R & McIvor A. *Lethal Work: A History of the Asbestos Tragedy in Scotland*. Tuckwell Press Ltd, East Lothian, 2000.

Peto J, Decarli A, La Vecchia C, Levi F & Negri E. The European mesothelioma epidemic. *British Journal of Cancer* 1999; **79**(3–4): 666–672.

Toms JR, ed. *CancerStats Monograph 2004*. Cancer Research UK, London, 2004.

Treasure T & Sedrakyan A. Pleural mesothelioma: little evidence, still time to do trials. *Lancet* 2004; **364**(9440): 1183–1185.

# CHAPTER 7

# Surgery for Non-Small Cell Lung Cancer

*Ian Hunt and Tom Treasure*

---

**OVERVIEW**

- Whether a lung cancer patient is a candidate for surgery depends on the type of cancer, the extent of the primary tumour, limited or absent spread to lymph nodes, and the absence of distant metastases.
- A histological diagnosis should be obtained whenever possible prior to operating.
- Staging is mandatory prior to any attempted surgical resection.
- Only a minority of patients with lung cancer are operated upon; however, surgical removal of the cancer when possible offers the best chance of a cure. It is for this reason that surgery comes ahead of radiotherapy and chemotherapy in the order of chapters in this book.

---

The question "Should this patient have an operation?" should be asked early in the assessment of each case. Only if the patient can be cured with an acceptably low risk of mortality and morbidity should we advise an operation. The assessment of the case should be structured to answer three questions:

1 Can the cancer be completely removed by operation?
2 Is the patient fit to undergo a chest operation?
3 Will the patient have enough lung function remaining to have a tolerable quality of life?

The questions can be answered in any order because a clear cut "no" to any one of the three is sufficient to preclude an operation (see Box 7.1).

Unless all of the cancer can be removed by the operation there is no gain in either length of life or in quality of life obtained by

---

Box 7.1 **Geographical variations in lung cancer operations**

Surgical resection rates for lung cancer vary geographically. The UK as a whole has a low rate of resection at around 13% compared to parts of Western Europe and the USA where it is about 25%. Reasons for this variation are likely to be multifactorial and to include later stage of presentation, more aggressive tumour types and higher co-morbidity.

---

*ABC of Lung Cancer.* Edited by I. Hunt, M. Muers and T. Treasure. © 2009 Blackwell Publishing, ISBN: 978-1-4051-4652-4.

surgery in our present state of knowledge. We must therefore establish the classification and the stage of the cancer.

## Classification of lung cancer suitable for operation

The classification of lung cancer depends upon the appearance of the cancer cells, as viewed by an expert pathologist looking down a microscope. At present we use a simple dichotomous classification into 'small cell' and 'non-small cell' lung cancer (SCLC and NSCLC). This arose because patients with small-cell cancers (previously known as oat cell cancer) who had operations intended to cure them, still died of their cancer; and they died about as soon as they would have done if the cancer had never been operated upon. This is because (with rare exceptions) even when the cancer looks curable, there are already microscopic deposits well beyond what can be removed surgically. When we started to use chemotherapy for lung cancer in the 1980s it was found that it was SCLC that most often responded and that sometimes the response was dramatic with significant tumour shrinkage. Chemotherapy rather than surgery has been advised for proven small-cell lung cancer (SCLC) since that time.

## Diagnosis of non-small cell lung cancer prior to surgery

Diagnostic methods include biopsy through the bronchoscope for central tumours and computed tomography (CT)-guided needle biopsy for peripheral tumours (see Chapter 4). On other occasions we may obtain tissue from metastatic deposits, in which case the cancer is by definition not operable.

In some instances investigations to obtain histology have failed to prove cancer but the suspicion of cancer is high based on clinical and radiological evidence. In that eventuality the patient's fitness for surgery is established and the stage of the cancer is determined on the presumption that it is NSCLC that we are dealing with. The diagnosis is confirmed by intraoperative biopsy with frozen section examination. This means that we have already performed a major operation (an incision in the chest called a thoracotomy) and it may turn out not to be cancer. Proceeding to major surgery with this uncertainty requires fully informed consent about the choices that might have to be made.

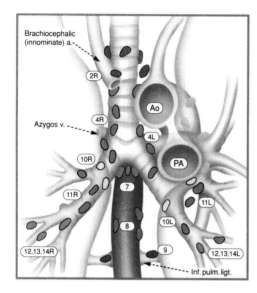

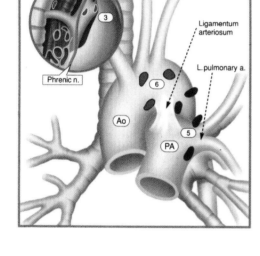

## Superior mediastinal nodes

● **1 Highest mediastinal**

● **2 Upper paratracheal**

● **3 Pre-vascular and retrotracheal**

● **4 Lowner paratracheal**
  **(including azygos nodes)**

$N_2$ = single digit, ipsilateral
$N_3$ = single digit, contralateral or supraclavicular

## Aortic nodes

● **5 Subaortic (A-P window)**

● **6 Para-aortic (ascending**
  **aorta or phrenic)**

## Inferior mediastinal nodes

● **7 Subcarinal**

● **8 Paraesophageal**
  **(below carina)**

● **9 Pulmonary ligament**

## $N_1$ nodes

○ **10 Hilar**

● **11 Intertobar**

● **12 Lobar**

● **13 Segmental**

● **14 Subsegmental**

**Figure 7.1** A regional lymph node map according to anatomical landmarks. (Reproduced with permission from Mountain & Dresler 1997.)

## Staging of non-small cell lung cancer suitable for surgery

In Chapter 4 we have described the criteria for staging NSCLC according to the tumour node metastasis (TNM) classification. To understand selection of cases for surgery it is easier to consider these in reverse order, as follows:

- **Metastases (M stage)**: almost without exception, metastases render the cancer beyond complete removal and therefore outside the realms of surgical cure. M1 therefore precludes surgery. Sometimes metastases are obvious and may be the reason for the original presentation, but we should actively exclude them by positron emission tomography (PET) scanning all potentially surgical patients. Patients with cancer suitable for surgery should be stage M0.
- **Lymph nodes (N stage)**: surgical cases should be stage N0 or N1. There is no evidence that we offer the patient any advantage whether in terms of survival or quality of life if we

attempt surgery when there is already spread to the mediastinal nodes or beyond. We use a combination of CT, PET and, where necessary, obtain a biopsy of mediastinal nodes to ensure that the cancer is not beyond the N0/1 stage. The regional lymph node map aids in identification and communication between the members of the multidisciplinary team (MDT) regarding N status (Figure 7.1).

- **Tumour (T stage)**: most surgical cases are T1 or T2. That means that all of the primary tumour can be removed with clear margins within an anatomical lung resection. Note though that a T2 tumour may be removed within a lobe but a T1 tumour may still require pneumonectomy, so the operation to resect the tumour requires specific surgical assessment. Surgical clearance may still be achievable with local extension into the chest wall (T3) and patients may be cured, but this requires careful surgical assessment. Although heroic resections of T4 tumours are described there is not good evidence that this is in the patient's best interest as virtually all recur (Figure 7.2).

| T/N | T1 | T2 | T3 | T4 |
|-----|-----|-----|-----|-----|
| N0 | IA | IB | IIB | IIIB |
| N1 | IIA | IIB | IIIA | IIIB |
| N2 | IIIA | IIIA | IIIA | IIIB |
| N3 | IIIB | IIIB | IIIB | IIIB |

**Figure 7.2** Lung cancer stages as derived from T (tumour) status and N (nodal) status. Cases in green boxes should be offered surgery with curative intent if sufficiently fit. Red boxes indicate cases where an operation is generally regarded as futile and to offer no survival advantage. Amber boxes indicate reasons for caution; these are cases where adjuvant chemotherapy may be considered, for example.

## Fitness for surgery on initial assessment

Lung cancer occurs with increasing frequency with age and predominately afflicts smokers or ex-smokers. An overall clinical assessment should be made before the patient is presented to the MDT (see Chapter 3). All patients being considered for lung resection should be directly questioned about exercise tolerance. Some of these patients are clearly unfit for anaesthesia, thoracotomy and the necessary lung resection right from the outset. They can be spared the inconvenience of assessments that are only relevant to candidates for surgery. On the other hand if the decision is marginal, work-up might include more rigorous cancer staging and detailed lung function tests aimed at specifically assessing whether they will tolerate the loss of lung tissue.

Provided careful assessment is made, for patients undergoing lung cancer surgery with clinical stage I–II disease, the outcomes are similar in the >70-year age group to the younger patient groups. Despite the curative intent of surgery, five-year survival for stage I and II disease still varies between 50 and 70%, with much of the subsequent mortality associated with disseminated disease unrecognised at initial surgery.

## Fitness for surgery after full assessment

If the cancer appears curable by surgery more detailed assessment of the patient's ability to withstand the necessary operation must be made. Will the loss of lung required to clear the cancer be tolerated? This goes beyond whether the patient is fit to withstand general anaesthesia.

Basic requirements are formal lung function tests using spirometry (Figure 7.3) including forced expiratory volume in the first second ($FEV_1$) and forced vital capacity (FVC) as well as diffusion capacity. The British Thoracic Society (BTS) guidelines suggest that for a patient to withstand a lobectomy or pneumonectomy without significant postoperative disability the post-bronchodilator $FEV_1$ should be >1.5 L and >2.0 L, respectively (Figure 7.4 and Box 7.2).

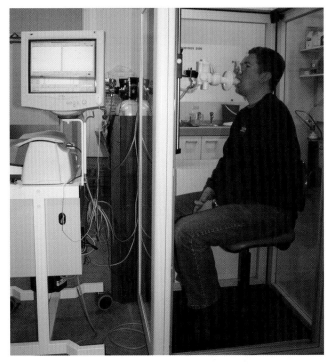

**Figure 7.3** Spirometry with flow volume loops to assess the mechanical properties of the respiratory system by measuring expiratory volumes and flow rates.

## The choice of surgical procedure

Surgery with curative intent requires the tumour to be localized or to have limited local–regional spread, which allows *en bloc* resection and removal of all the primary cancer and the regional lymph nodes.

## Standard major pulmonary resection

Full anatomic resection is defined as a resection of either a complete lobe of the lung (lobectomy) or the entire lung (pneumonectomy) and requires dissection and division of hilar vessels and bronchial structures (Figure 7.5).

Lobectomy is the procedure of choice for patients with stage I and II NSCLC who can tolerate the loss of lung required. The standard operation is performed through a posterolateral thoracotomy (Figure 7.6). The segmental arteries, lobar bronchus and draining pulmonary veins are dissected and divided, and the bronchus is usually stapled. In hospital, mortality following standard lobectomy is 2–3%. Chest drains are left until any air leak has ceased. The mediastinum, diaphragm and the lung conform to each other and the postoperative X-ray can be near normal in appearance (Figure 7.7).

Removal of a whole lung (pneumonectomy) is less frequently performed. It is indicated if the tumour is centrally placed, involves the main bronchus or pulmonary artery, or is straddling the major fissure. In hospital, mortality following pneumonectomy is of the order of 10%, so even more rigorous assessment for fitness for surgery and prediction of ability to function after the lung is removed

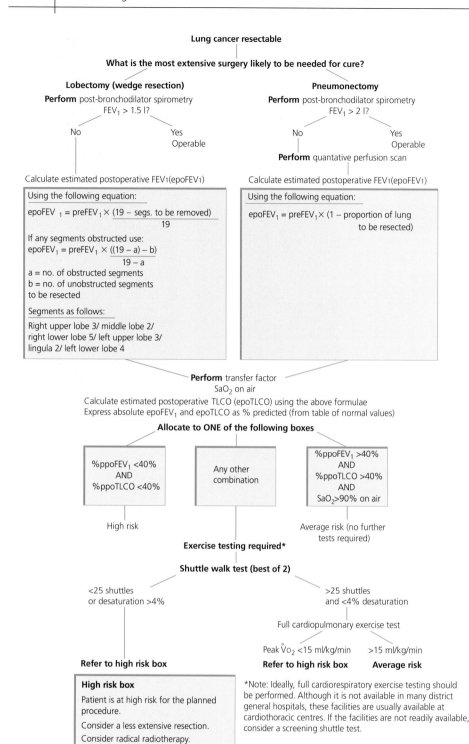

**Lung cancer resectable**

**What is the most extensive surgery likely to be needed for cure?**

**Lobectomy (wedge resection)**

**Perform** post-bronchodilator spirometry
$FEV_1 > 1.5$ l?

No → → Yes
Operable

Calculate estimated postoperative FEV1(epoFEV1)

Using the following equation:

$$epoFEV_1 = preFEV_1 \times \frac{(19 - segs. \text{ to be removed})}{19}$$

If any segments obstructed use:
$$epoFEV_1 = preFEV_1 \times \frac{((19 - a) - b)}{19 - a}$$

a = no. of obstructed segments
b = no. of unobstructed segments
to be resected

Segments as follows:

Right upper lobe 3/ middle lobe 2/
right lower lobe 5/ left upper lobe 3/
lingula 2/ left lower lobe 4

**Pneumonectomy**

**Perform** post-bronchodilator spirometry
$FEV_1 > 2$ l?

No → → Yes
Operable

**Perform** quantative perfusion scan

Calculate estimated postoperative FEV1(epoFEV1)

Using the following equation:

$$epoFEV_1 = preFEV_1 \times (1 - \text{proportion of lung to be resected})$$

**Perform** transfer factor
$SaO_2$ on air
Calculate estimated postoperative TLCO (epoTLCO) using the above formulae
Express absolute $epoFEV_1$ and epoTLCO as % predicted (from table of normal values)

**Allocate to ONE of the following boxes**

%ppoFEV$_1$ <40%
AND
%ppoTLCO <40%

Any other
combination

%ppoFEV$_1$ >40%
AND
%ppoTLCO >40%
AND
$SaO_2$>90% on air

High risk

Average risk (no further
tests required)

**Exercise testing required***

**Shuttle walk test (best of 2)**

<25 shuttles
or desaturation >4%

>25 shuttles
and <4% desaturation

Full cardiopulmonary exercise test

Peak $\overset{\circ}{V}O_2$ <15 ml/kg/min        >15 ml/kg/min

**Refer to high risk box**          **Refer to high risk box**    **Average risk**

**High risk box**

Patient is at high risk for the planned
procedure.

Consider a less extensive resection.

Consider radical radiotherapy.

*Note: Ideally, full cardiorespiratory exercise testing should
be performed. Although it is not available in many district
general hospitals, these facilities are usually available at
cardiothoracic centres. If the facilities are not readily available,
consider a screening shuttle test.

**Figure 7.4** An algorithm for the selection of
patients for resection for lung cancer. $FEV_1$,
forced expiratory volume in one second; FVC,
forced vital capacity; TLCO, carbon monoxide
transfer factor (Reproduced with permission
from Armstrong *et al.* 2001).

is mandatory if the patient is to tolerate this procedure. Following removal of the lung the intrathoracic air space remaining is gradually replaced by fluid as the air is absorbed (Figure 7.8). The most serious complications of pneumonectomy are breakdown of the bronchial closure and infection of the pneumonectomy space (bronchopleural fistula).

## Sublobar resection

Wedge resection refers to the removal of a non-anatomical portion of the lung, usually performed as removal of a 'wedge' of parenchyma with a tumour near the pleural surface. Wedge resection can be undertaken using a 'keyhole approach' with thoracoscopic surgery (Figure 7.9), thus sparing the patient a chest wall incision as well as reducing to a minimum the loss of the lung.

Segmentectomy is an anatomic resection of a bronchopulmonary segment. Both of these limited resections involve division of the lung parenchyma, which increases the risk of local recurrence. This procedure has a role in patients who can only tolerate very limited lung resection due to presence of comorbidity or pulmonary compromise.

---

Box 7.2 **Workup surgery in patients with potentially curable lung cancer**

There should be formal liaison in borderline cases between the referring chest physician and the thoracic surgical team. If not clearly operable following spirometry, further pulmonary tests including estimation of carbon monoxide transfer factor (TLCO) if not already performed, resting oxygen saturation, isotope or ventilation/perfusion (V/Q) scans, and even full cardiopulmonary exercise tests are performed to help with further analysis. Patients will accept risk in exchange for a chance of cure, so the lowest possible mortality may protect the surgical figures but is not in the best interest of cancer patients as a whole. These judgements must be made explicitly and shared honestly with the patient.

---

## Extended resection

Extensive metastases to mediastinal lymph nodes and beyond precludes surgical cure. On the other hand, local invasion may not.

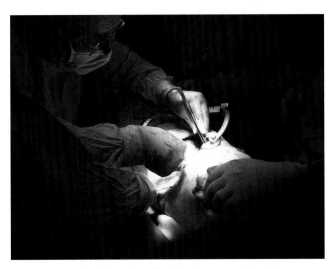

**Figure 7.6** A patient in lateral position showing a posterolateral thoracotomy incision.

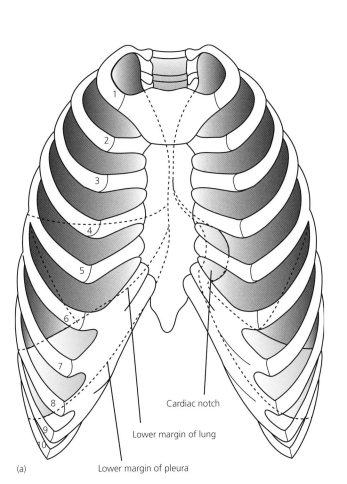

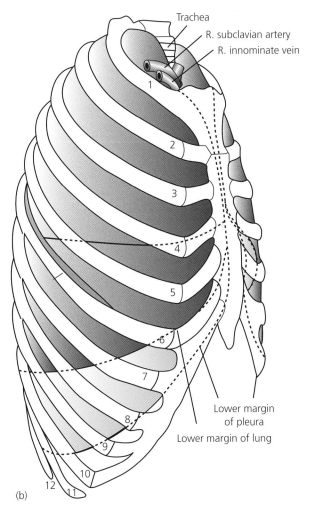

**Figure 7.5** (a) and (b) Diagrams of the lung and its lobes. (Reproduced with permission from *Gray's Anatomy of the Human Body*.)

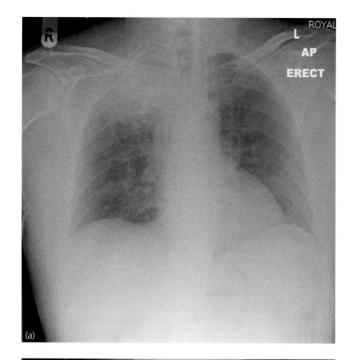

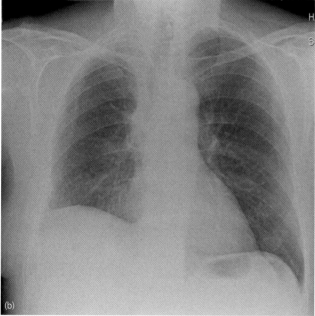

**Figure 7.7** Chest X-ray (CXR) pre (a) and post (b) right upper lobectomy demonstrating how the remaining structures 'fill' the space left by the excised upper lobe.

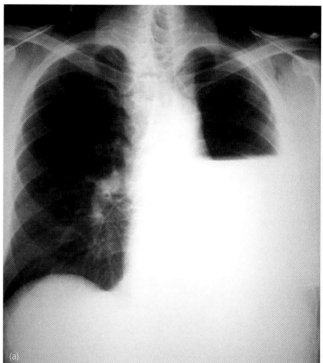

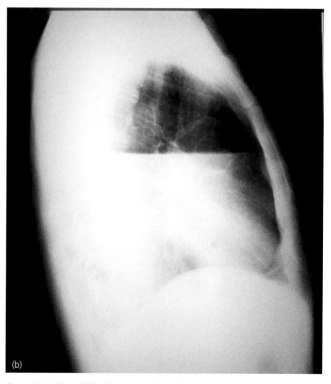

**Figure 7.8** (a) and (b) Chest X-rays (CXR) following left pneumonectomy with air-fluid levels clearly seen.

Lung resection may be combined with limited chest wall resection or reconstruction of the proximal airways in exceptional cases to obtain surgical clearance.

## Minimally invasive thorascopic resection

The advent of minimally invasive or 'keyhole' video-assisted thorascopic surgery (VATS) has significantly altered the surgical management of certain thoracic conditions, most notably in the tissue diagnosis of the solitary or indeterminate pulmonary nodule (Figure 7.9). Beyond lung biopsies and wedge resections, full anatomical resections are currently performed uncommonly but survival data suggest similar outcomes and probably fewer complications than with thoracotomy. Mediastinal lymph

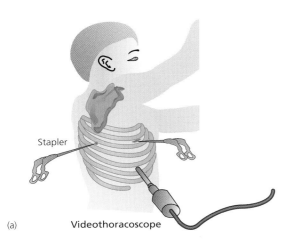

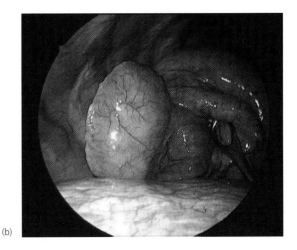

**Figure 7.9** (a) A video-assisted thorascopic surgery (VATS) image showing port positions allowing surgeon to resect tumour; one of the ports is for a camera. (b) An intraoperative thorascopic image.

nodes are routinely sampled or sometimes cleared for complete pathological (termed pTNM) staging.

## Postoperative care

Patients are encouraged to breath and therefore have the endotracheal tube removed soon after the procedure; positive pressure ventilation is avoided. Intensive care with the implication of elective ventilation is also best avoided, but care should routinely be provided in a high-dependency unit (HDU).

Good pain management in the postoperative period is critical to recovery. Thoracic epidural or paravertebral anaesthesia is standard, as is intravenous patient-controlled analgesia (PCA) (see Chapter 8, Figure 8.8). These allow deep breathing and coughing. Early and repeated chest physiotherapy is used to pre-empt the complications of retained secretions, atelectasis and chest infection. Early mobilisation physiotherapy is encouraged, and patients generally leave hospital in five to ten days (Figure 7.10).

## Further reading

Armstrong P, Congleton J, Fountain SW, *et al.* British Thoracic Society guidelines on the selection of patients with lung cancer for surgery. British Thoracic Society and Society of Cardiothoracic Surgeons of Great Britain and Ireland Working Party. *Thorax* 2001; **56**: 89–108.

*Gray's Anatomy of the Human Body.* www.bartleby.com/107.

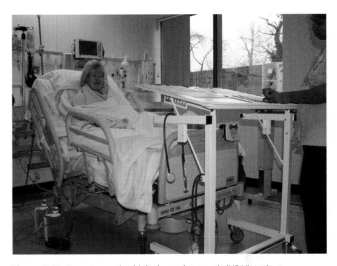

**Figure 7.10** A postoperative high-dependency unit (HDU) patient.

Mountain CF & Dresler CM. Regional lymph node classification for lung cancer staging. *Chest* 1997; **111**: 1718–1723.

NICE. *Referral Guidelines for Suspected Cancer.* NICE Clinical Guideline No. 27. National Institute for Health & Clinical Excellence, London 2005: http://www.nice.org.uk.

Shields TW, LoCicero J III, Ponn RB & Rusch VW, eds. *General Thoracic Surgery* 6th edition. Lippincott Williams & Wilkins, Philadelphia, 2004.

Treasure T, Hunt I, Keogh B & Pagano D, eds. *The Evidence for Cardiothoracic Surgery.* tfm publishing, Shrewsbury, 2004.

# CHAPTER 8

# Radiotherapy for Non-Small Cell Lung Cancer

*Jeanette Dickson and Michael Snee*

**OVERVIEW**

- Radiotherapy is the most commonly used treatment modality in Non-Small Cell Lung Cancer (NSCLC).
- Radiotherapy can be used with curative or palliative intent.
- Side-effects associated with radiotherapy can occur around the time treatment is delivered (acute) or after many months or sometimes years (late).
- Radiotherapy is delivered using linear accelerators (LINAC), which need to be housed in purpose-built facilities. Therefore, patients will often need to travel to a radiotherapy centre for treatment.

Radiotherapy is the commonest treatment modality for NSCLC with more than 50% of patients receiving this at some point in their illness. Radiotherapy involves the accurate delivery of high-energy photon (X-ray) beams targeted at a cancer. These beams are generated using electricity by a purpose-built machine, termed a linear accelerator (LINAC; Figure 8.1). Radiotherapy can be given with curative (radical) or palliative intent.

## Mechanism of action

At a cellular level the photon beam causes the formation of free radicals that interact with DNA causing damage. If the cell is able to repair the damage then it will be resistant to radiotherapy and survive. Cells that succumb to lethal radiation damage die by apoptosis and are removed by the body's normal mechanisms. Thus, radiation side-effects are the consequence of radiation damage to normal tissues surrounding the cancer.

## Tumour radiobiology

The probability of cure, termed tumour control probability (TCP), and the incidence of side-effects are both dependant on a number of factors: these are the total dose delivered (in grays), the dose delivered per fraction, and in some cancers including NSCLC the

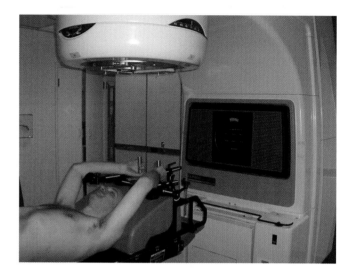

**Figure 8.1** A linear accelerator (LINAC).

overall treatment time (in days). Courses of radical radiotherapy are conventionally delivered in daily fractions (Monday–Friday) for four to six weeks. Increasing the total dose delivered increases the TCP. However, if the dose per fraction is kept constant this increases overall treatment duration, which decreases the TCP. Decreasing overall treatment time (acceleration) improves TCP, but if acceleration is achieved by increasing dose per fraction the risk of late radiation side-effects is increased. There has been a lot of research into altered fractionation schedules (hyperfractionation; i.e. more than one treatment per day), which leaves the risk of late radiation side-effects constant but significantly accelerates the treatment delivery time. However, significant time (six hours) must be left in between each fraction to allow for normal tissue repair. In the 1990s continuous hyperfractionated accelerated radiotherapy (CHART) was developed, which delivers radiotherapy three times per day with a six-hour interfraction interval, for twelve consecutive days. In a randomised study three-year survival following CHART was found to be 10% higher than conventional treatment. However, staffing issues over evening and weekend treatment and scepticism about the radiation dose used in the control arm has lead to limited adoption of this schedule, despite its incorporation into NICE guidelines (NICE, 2005; Table 8.1).

*ABC of Lung Cancer.* Edited by I. Hunt, M. Muers and T. Treasure. © 2009 Blackwell Publishing, ISBN: 978-1-4051-4652-4.

**Table 8.1** Comparison of different radiotherapy regimens.

|  | Chart | Acceleration | Conventional |
|---|---|---|---|
| Total dose (Gy) | 54 | 55 | 64 |
| Overall treatment time (days) | 12 | 28 | 44 |
| Dose per fraction (Gy) | 1.5 | 2.75 | 2 |
| Biological equivalent dose (At 2 Gy /#) | 63 | 63 | 64 |

Box 8.1 **Assessment prior to radiotherapy treatment**

Patients treated radically should have a combined positron emission tomography and computed tomography (PET-CT) scan and full lung function tests, as well as being able to lie flat and still for five minutes.

A similar improvement in survival to that seen in the CHART study has been seen when radiotherapy is given concurrently with chemotherapy (chemo-irradiation). Chemotherapy can potentiate the side-effects of radiotherapy when delivered concurrently, leading to an increased risk of both acute and late toxicity. However, the fact that the control arms of such studies used inadequate doses and/or suboptimal techniques has lead to controversy over the best method to adopt. This is an area of ongoing study internationally.

## Radical radiotherapy planning

Radical radiotherapy, where the aim is to cure, is utilised in two groups of patients. The first includes patients that have a tumour that is technically resectable but surgery is deemed too risky because of respiratory or cardiovascular comorbidity. The second group includes patients that are generally fit but that have locally advanced disease that is unresectable (generally either stage T4 or N2). All patients treated with radical intent require careful work-up prior to embarking on the treatment planning process. Ideally all patients should have a combined positron emission tomography and computed tomography (PET-CT) scan and full lung function, including carbon monoxide transfer factor (TLCO), measured. Some patients with severe impairment of lung function will be unsuitable for both radical radiotherapy and surgery (see Box 8.1).

Patients then undergo a planning CT scan in the treatment position. They lie completely supine on a rigid, flat (rather than cupped) couch. Permanent skin marks allow reproducible patient set-up on a daily basis. The patients' arms are usually raised above the head on a customised immobilisation device. This allows the treatment to be delivered from a greater number of directions. Thus, patients with severe osteoporosis, congestive cardiac failure or joint problems may be unsuitable for treatment (Figure 8.2).

All visible cancer is outlined on the computerised planning system by the clinical oncologist, using information from the

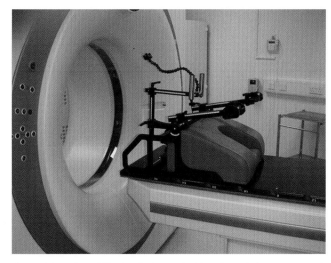

**Figure 8.2** An immobilisation device used with patients during a computed tomography (CT) planning scan.

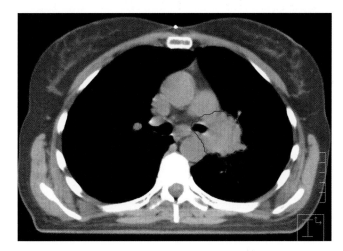

**Figure 8.3** A left central tumour with gross tumour volume (GTV) outlined in red.

bronchoscopy as well as imaging studies. This is known as the gross tumour volume (GTV; Figure 8.3). The GTV is grown using a three-dimensional computer algorithm in all directions to account for microscopic spread, patient movement during treatment and organ motion during breathing. The resulting volume is known as the planning target volume (PTV; Figure 8.4). Dedicated planning physicists then produce an individualised treatment plan, which optimises radiotherapy delivery to the cancer while minimising the dose to the critical normal structures of the lungs and spinal cord (Figure 8.5). Radical treatment is delivered via a number (usually three or four) of radiation beams. These are shaped in the machine head by multileaf collimators (MLC; Figure 8.6). This reduces the volume of normal tissue irradiated, thus limiting treatment-related side-effects and damage. Each fraction of radiotherapy takes about three minutes to deliver. Accurate patient positioning on the treatment machine means that the patient is in the treatment room for about ten minutes.

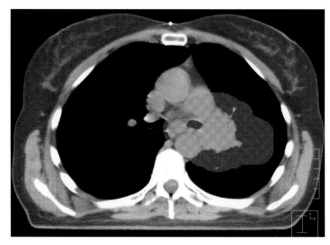

**Figure 8.4** A planning target volume (PTV) grown geometrically using a computer algorithm.

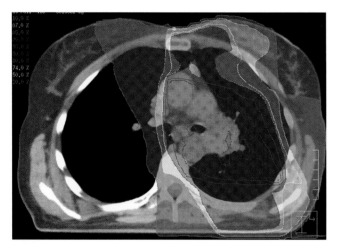

**Figure 8.5** Dose distribution of radiation in patients in planning field.

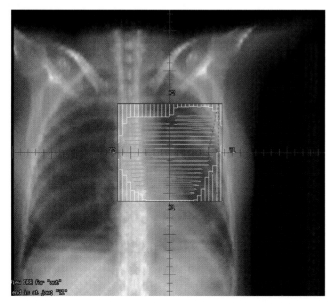

**Figure 8.6** An anterior treatment field shaped by multileaf collimators (MLC).

## Palliative radiotherapy planning

The aim of palliative radiotherapy is to produce the maximum symptomatic benefit with the least side-effects in the quickest possible time. In the 1980s and 1990s there were a number of Medical Research Council (MRC) studies that defined palliative thoracic radiotherapy in the UK. These trials compared the benefit derived from a number of different treatment schedules with the side-effects experienced, recorded from both the physician's and patient's point of view.

In patients with poor performance status, one or two fractions (treatments) of radiotherapy gave as good palliation (both in terms of effect and duration) as a two-week treatment schedule. In patients of good performance status and with locally advanced disease that was too large for radical radiotherapy, a daily fractionation schedule of 12–13 treatments gave a survival benefit comparable to that achieved with chemotherapy in advanced disease. The cost to the patient was a slight increase in acute radiation side-effects.

Palliative radiotherapy is administered using a simple technique that usually allows the treatment to be delivered on the same day. The disease is treated using two fields applied in opposite directions (anterior and posterior). Thus, a whole block of tissue can be irradiated in continuity. Technological advances have allowed the development of virtual simulation, which combines a CT scan with the planning computer allowing direct placement of palliative fields whilst visualising the disease three-dimensionally. This can reduce field size, which in turn reduces treatment-related toxicity.

## Radiotherapy side-effects

Acute radiation side-effects occur around the time treatment is given. In palliative treatments they last for a few days to a week or two. For radical treatment courses they last for 4–6 weeks following the end of treatment. They occur due to cell depletion in rapidly dividing tissues within the radiotherapy field, e.g. skin and oesophageal mucosa. The most commonly occurring local side-effects of thoracic radiotherapy are skin erythema, oesophagitis (if the mediastinum is included in the radiotherapy field) and cough. Acute side-effects are self-limiting and thus simple supportive measures in addition to patient education are usually all that is required. Systemic side-effects of radiotherapy treatment are thought to arise due to cytokine release from cells, especially white blood cells, within the radiotherapy field. They commonly manifest as tiredness and lethargy. Patients will occasionally report rigors and a 'flu-like' syndrome that is short lived in duration (hours).

Late radiation side-effects do not arise within six months of treatment, but can potentially develop at any time thereafter. As the median survival of NSCLC patients is less than a year they are rarely seen in the palliative setting. However, when treatment is given with radical (curative) intent it is extremely important to minimize the risk of late side-effects as once they become established they are irreversible and can have serious functional implications. They occur due to two main factors. First, there is depletion of stem cells in slowly dividing tissues, e.g. lung and spinal cord. Second, the vascular damage caused by radiotherapy

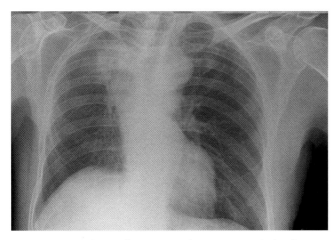

**Figure 8.7** Late radiation effects: CXR/CT demonstrating RT-induced changes.

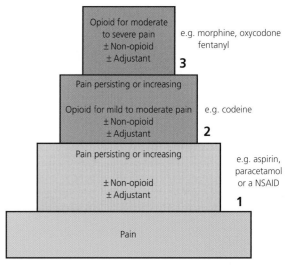

**Figure 8.8** The concept of the analgesic ladder is applicable for different lung cancer treatments including radiotherapy and surgery. NSAID, non-steroidal anti-inflammatory drug.

can lead to significant tissue ischaemia and scarring, which can make the problem progressive. The risk of developing late radiation-induced side-effects is the main factor limiting the dose of radiation that can be safely delivered in the radical setting. Pneumonitis and lung fibrosis after radiotherapy leads to loss of lung function and breathlessness (Figure 8.7). Damage to the spinal cord leads to radiation myelitis; in the worse-case scenario this can lead to paralysis. With technological advances in treatment planning this is now virtually never seen.

## Treatment of radiation side-effects

Patients can wash normally during radiotherapy but should avoid scented soap and prolonged immersion in the bath. Unguents such as aqueous cream applied twice daily can minimize skin irritation. Codeine linctus can be used as a suppressant in cases of troublesome cough, and this can provide an additional analgesic effect in oesophagitis. Soluble analgesics escalating, as required, up the World Health Organisation (WHO) ladder can be given for oesophagitis (Figure 8.8) and liquid antacids can be taken approximately 30 minutes prior to eating. Following radical radiotherapy it is occasionally necessary to prescribe opioid analgesia and liquid food supplements; dietetic input can be a very helpful adjunct in this situation. Smoking exacerbates acute radiation reactions and should be discouraged, especially in those receiving treatment with curative intent.

## Radiotherapy outcomes

Radical radiotherapy is delivered by a complex technical process that requires significant input from non-medical team members such as physicists and radiographers. It is an invaluable treatment in the palliation of symptoms associated with lung cancer. In those patients with only locally advanced disease and with good performance status, high-dose palliative radiotherapy provides an identical survival benefit to palliative chemotherapy. In those with poor performance status, palliative radiotherapy can improve intrathoracic symptoms in a much shorter time period than chemotherapy. This is especially true in the case of haemoptysis, which many patients find a distressing visible sign of their terminal disease.

## Further reading

Hoskin PJ, ed. *Radiotherapy in Practice: External Beam Therapy.* Oxford University Press, New York, 2006.

Lester JF, Macbeth FR, Toy E & Coles B. Palliative radiotherapy regimens for non-small cell lung cancer. *Cochrane Database of Systematic Reviews* 2006, Issue 3. Art. No.: CD002143. DOI: 10.1002/14651858.CD002143.pub2: http://www.cochrane.org/reviews/en/ab002143.htm.

Neal AJ & Hoskin PJ, eds. *Clinical Oncology: Basic Principles and Practice*, 3rd edition. Hodder Arnold, London, 2003.

NICE. *Referral Guidelines for Suspected Cancer.* NICE Clinical Guideline No. 27. National Institute for Health & Clinical Excellence, London 2005: http://www.nice.org.uk.

Saunders M, Dische S, Barrett A, Harvey A, Gibson D & Parmar M. Continuous hyperfractionated accelerated radiotherapy (CHART) versus conventional radiotherapy in non-small cell lung cancer: a randomised multicentre trial. *Lancet* 1997; **350**: 161–165.

# CHAPTER 9

# Combination Therapies for Lung Cancer

*Penella Woll, Sally Moore and Ian Hunt*

## OVERVIEW

- Different combinations of surgery, radiotherapy and chemotherapy can be given at varying stages of disease.
- Postoperative radiotherapy is not recommended following complete surgical excision.
- Preoperative radiotherapy is not recommended.
- In patients with early-stage disease, chemotherapy can be combined with surgery by giving it either before (neoadjuvant) or after (adjuvant) surgery.
- Postoperative adjuvant chemotherapy can improve survival following complete surgical resection.
- Preoperative neoadjuvant chemotherapy is not routinely recommended.
- In locally advanced disease, combination chemoradiotherapy is the treatment of choice in appropriate patients.

In lung cancer, as in other tumour types, combining different treatment modalities can be more successful than treatment with a single modality. Various combinations of surgery, radiotherapy and chemotherapy are useful in different stages of disease. Current research is investigating the role of biologically-targeted agents combined with these.

## Early-stage disease

For the minority of patients diagnosed with NSCLC at an early enough stage, surgery offers the best chance of cure. However, even the few patients with stage Ia disease (T1 N0 M0) have only a 60–70% chance of surviving five years; for those with stage Ib disease (T2 N0 M0) this figure is only 40%. The prognosis for other operable patients is worse (Figure 9.1). Most patients who die following lung cancer recurrence after surgical resection do so from distant metastases (Figures 9.2 and 9.3). There is clearly scope for improvement.

## Surgery and radiotherapy

It was hoped that combining surgery and radiotherapy would improve cure rates by reducing local recurrence. Preoperative radiotherapy might also reduce dissemination of tumour cells at the time of resection. It remains unclear which lung cancer patients can benefit from combining surgery and radiotherapy.

### Postoperative radiotherapy

A Cochrane review known as the postoperative radiotherapy (PORT) meta-analysis included nine studies of surgery with or without radiotherapy for NSCLC, involving over 2000 patients (PORT Meta-Analysis Trialists Group 2003). Overall, patients who received postoperative radiotherapy had a worse survival rate than those who had surgery alone, with the proportion alive at two years reduced from 55 to 48%. Most of the studies used outdated radiotherapy techniques that carried a greater risk of later heart problems than encountered with modern methods. Adjuvant radiotherapy is therefore not recommended following complete surgical excision. However, where the surgical excision is incomplete, the risk of local tumour recurrence is very high, and postoperative radiotherapy may be offered. A new European trial is planned that will test the use of modern radiotherapy techniques in patients at high risk of local disease recurrence because of lymph node involvement.

### Preoperative radiotherapy

Preoperative radiotherapy has not been shown to offer any benefits over surgery alone and is not recommended.

## Surgery and chemotherapy

In many tumour types, including breast cancer, colorectal cancer and osteosarcoma, the addition of 'adjuvant' chemotherapy to surgery improves the chance of long-term survival and is routinely recommended in the management of primary disease. Following surgery for lung cancer many patients relapse and die with widespread 'systemic' disease. Early systemic treatment offers the opportunity to treat micrometastases, which are much more chemosensitive than established secondary tumours. Preoperative (neoadjuvant) chemotherapy tackles micrometastases early and may shrink the primary tumour prior to surgery, but is

*ABC of Lung Cancer*. Edited by I. Hunt, M. Muers and T. Treasure. © 2009 Blackwell Publishing, ISBN: 978-1-4051-4652-4.

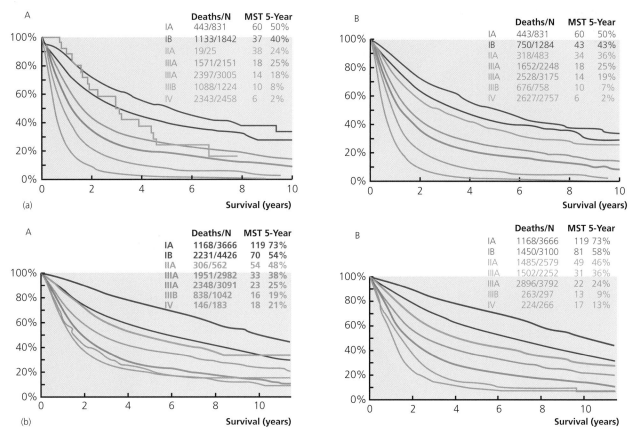

| | Deaths/N | MST | 5-Year |
|---|---|---|---|
| IA | 443/831 | 60 | 50% |
| IB | 1133/1842 | 37 | 40% |
| IIA | 19/25 | 38 | 24% |
| IIIA | 1571/2151 | 18 | 25% |
| IIIA | 2397/3005 | 14 | 18% |
| IIIB | 1088/1224 | 10 | 8% |
| IV | 2343/2458 | 6 | 2% |

| | Deaths/N | MST | 5-Year |
|---|---|---|---|
| IA | 443/831 | 60 | 50% |
| IB | 750/1284 | 43 | 43% |
| IIA | 318/483 | 34 | 36% |
| IIIA | 1652/2248 | 18 | 25% |
| IIIA | 2528/3175 | 14 | 19% |
| IIIB | 676/758 | 10 | 7% |
| IV | 2627/2757 | 6 | 2% |

| | Deaths/N | MST | 5-Year |
|---|---|---|---|
| IA | 1168/3666 | 119 | 73% |
| IB | 2231/4426 | 70 | 54% |
| IIA | 306/562 | 54 | 48% |
| IIIA | 1951/2982 | 33 | 38% |
| IIIA | 2348/3091 | 23 | 25% |
| IIIB | 838/1042 | 16 | 19% |
| IV | 146/183 | 18 | 21% |

| | Deaths/N | MST | 5-Year |
|---|---|---|---|
| IA | 1168/3666 | 119 | 73% |
| IB | 1450/3100 | 81 | 58% |
| IIA | 1485/2579 | 49 | 46% |
| IIIA | 1502/2252 | 31 | 36% |
| IIIA | 2896/3792 | 22 | 24% |
| IIIB | 263/297 | 13 | 9% |
| IV | 224/266 | 17 | 13% |

**Figure 9.1** Overall and five-year survival by clinical (a) and pathological (b) stage for patients with non-small cell lung cancer (NSCLC). MST, median survival time. (Reproduced with permission from Goldstraw *et al.* 2007.)

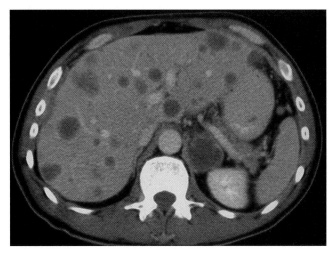

**Figure 9.2** A computed tomography (CT) scan demonstrating liver metastases.

associated with an increased risk of perioperative morbidity. Postoperative (adjuvant) chemotherapy does not delay or increase the risk of surgery, but the start of systemic treatment (and the chance of benefit) may be delayed if recovery from surgery is slow or complicated.

## Postoperative adjuvant chemotherapy

There is now compelling evidence from numerous randomised controlled trials (RCT) that postoperative adjuvant chemotherapy can improve the chance of survival of patients with completely resected NSCLC. A recent meta-analysis included data from 988 patients in seven RCT. Preoperative chemotherapy improved survival to an absolute benefit of 6%, increasing overall survival across all stages of disease from 14 to 20% at five years. Such modest improvements in survival may not seem dramatic, but it is clear from experience in other tumour types that many patients will feel that this is worthwhile. The majority of operated patients should therefore have the opportunity to discuss adjuvant chemotherapy with an oncologist. However, not all patients will be fit enough to consider cisplatin-based chemotherapy immediately after a thoracotomy, and about one-third of patients will accept adjuvant chemotherapy.

## Preoperative neoadjuvant chemotherapy

Two small-randomised studies of neoadjuvant chemotherapy, each enrolling just 60 patients, were reported in 1994. Both appeared to show that the survival of patients with stage IIIa NSCLC undergoing surgery could be substantially improved with preoperative chemotherapy (Figure 9.5). These results caused a huge amount of interest, and several larger studies were then set up to determine if these

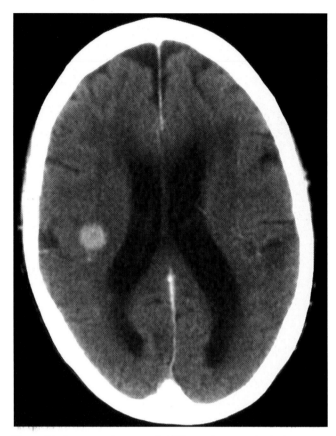

**Figure 9.3** A computed tomography (CT) scan demonstrating brain metastases.

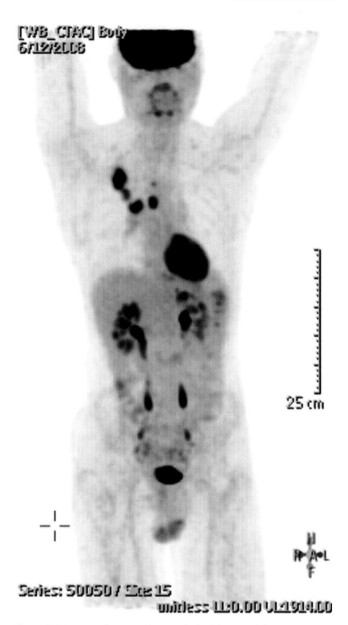

**Figure 9.4** PET scan demonstrating uptake in right upper lobe tumour, in right hilar and paratracheal lymph nodes consistent with N2 disease.

results could be reproduced. Two (from France and the UK) have now been reported. Neither showed a survival advantage for neoadjuvant chemotherapy. Importantly, very few tumours progressed during the chemotherapy and there was no increase in surgical complications subsequently. However, an updated meta-analysis including data from 1507 patients in eight RCT showed a small benefit for neoadjuvant chemotherapy. This is equivalent to an absolute survival benefit of 5% at five years. Neoadjuvant chemotherapy is therefore not routinely recommended.

## Locally advanced disease

Patients with hilar lymph node involvement or locally infiltrative tumours (stage IIIa or IIIb) (Figure 9.4) might be unsuitable for surgery, but some can be treated with radical radiotherapy. This treatment is described in Chapter 8. Although a small proportion of patients will have prolonged survival after such treatment, for the majority the outlook is dismal (Figure 9.1). There has therefore been interest in combining chemotherapy and radiotherapy to improve outcomes and there is now clear evidence that chemoradiotherapy results in better survival than radiotherapy alone for these patients. In addition to stage of disease, performance status is a major prognostic factor in this setting, with fitter patients deriving the most benefit. However, controversy remains about the best way to schedule these treatments.

### Sequential chemoradiotherapy

Seven randomised trials including nearly 2000 patients have compared outcomes in patients receiving radiotherapy alone or cisplatin-based chemotherapy followed by radiotherapy. All the patients had to be suitable for radical radiotherapy at presentation. There was a trend towards better response rates in the chemoradiotherapy arms, and survival was significantly better, with no difference in radiation toxicities.

### Concurrent chemoradiotherapy

Fourteen randomised trials, including 2400 patients have compared outcomes in patients receiving radiotherapy alone or concurrent chemoradiotherapy. Once again, chemoradiotherapy resulted in a reduced risk of death at two years and

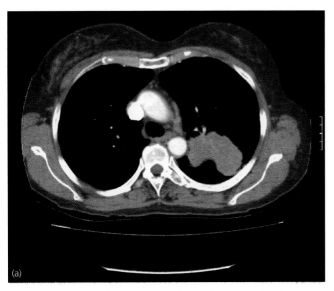
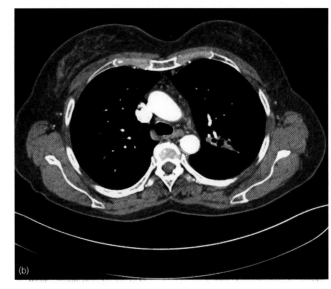

**Figure 9.5** A computed tomography (CT) scan of a tumour showing size pre- (a) and post-chemotherapy (b), prior to resection.

better progression-free survival. However, the risks of toxicity are greater when chemotherapy and radiotherapy are given concurrently. Three studies have compared sequential with concurrent chemoradiotherapy, and their early results suggest that concurrent treatment offers a survival advantage, but at the risk of worse toxicity.

## Primary chemotherapy for locally advanced non-small cell lung cancer

Patients with inoperable locally advanced NSCLC sometimes have disease that cannot be encompassed by a radical radiotherapy field. They are therefore unsuitable for planned chemoradiotherapy and the appropriate treatment is palliative chemotherapy. A proportion, however, might become eligible for radical local treatment (surgery or radiotherapy) if they have a dramatic response to primary chemotherapy (Figure 9.5). No studies have been carried out to date to determine whether local treatments prolong survival in this setting. However, a recent study randomised responding patients to surgery or radiotherapy and showed that radiotherapy was at least as good as surgery.

The role of combination therapies in managing patients with lung cancer is likely to expand as our understanding of lung cancer advances and new agents become available. Novel treatments including biologically-targeted agents (e.g. bevacizumab, erlotinib) and vaccines are currently being tested in combination with conventional treatment modalities.

## Further reading

Bradbury PA, Shepherd FA, Gilligan D, *et al.* Preoperative chemotherapy in patients with resectable non-small cell lung cancer: results of the MRC LU22/NVALT 2/EORTC 08012 multicentre randomised trial and update of systematic review. *Lancet* 2007; **369**: 1929–1937.

Burdett S, Stewart LA & Rydzeweska L. A systematic review and meta-analysis of the literature: chemotherapy and surgery versus surgery alone in non-small cell lung cancer. *Journal of Thoracic Oncology* 2006; **1**: 611–621.

PORT Meta-Analysis Trialists Group. Postoperative radiotherapy in non-small cell lung cancer. *Cochrane Database of Systematic Reviews* 2003; **1**: CD002142: http://www.cochrane.org.

Goldstraw P, Crowley J, Chansky K *et al.* The IASLC Lung Cancer Staging Project: proposals for the revision of the TNM stage groupings in the forthcoming (seventh) edition of the TNM Classification of Malignant Tumours. *Journal of Thoracic Oncology* 2007; **2**(8): 706–714.

Sedrakyan A, van Der Meulen J, O'Byrne K, Prendiville J, Hill J & Treasure T. Postoperative chemotherapy for non-small cell lung cancer: a systematic review and meta-analysis. *Journal of Thoracic and Cardiovascular Surgery* 2004; 128: 414–419.

# CHAPTER 10

# Screening for Lung Cancer

*Ian Hunt, Fergus Gleeson and Jenny Hill*

---

**OVERVIEW**

- Screening is the deliberate detection of disease before symptoms develop.
- A disease must fulfil certain criteria if a screening test is to have any benefit.
- Studies of lung cancer screening with chest X-ray (CXR) and sputum cytology have failed to demonstrate a reduction in lung cancer mortality.
- Evaluation of low-dose computed tomography (CT) and 'biomarkers' as a screening test for lung cancer is currently underway.
- No screening test has been shown to alter lung cancer mortality outcomes.
- Currently no international guidelines are recommending lung cancer screening in high-risk populations.

---

Box 10.1 **Criteria for a disease to be deemed appropriate for screening**

- There must be sufficient disease burden in the population.
- There must be an intervention available to positively affect the natural course of the disease.
- The screening test must have few false-positive results.
- The test must be acceptable to the patient.
- The programme should be cost-effective.

---

Screening is the deliberate detection of disease before symptoms develop when the disease is in its preclinical stage. To be of value, screening has to be sensitive enough to detect nearly all patients with disease at this early stage and to positively affect the usual outcome. To do this, the screening test must also correctly identify those without the disease and to be cost-effective (Box 10.1).

## Assessment of a screening programme: types of study

The idea of screening for lung cancer is not new, and dates back to when the first link between lung cancer and smoking was discovered in the 1950s (see Chapter 1). Lung cancer continues to claim around 33,000 lives a year in the UK and thus to impose a significant disease burden.

Screening programmes have focused on the evaluation of asymptomatic individuals believed to be at high risk for lung cancer. In assessing such programmes several research methods can be applied, with the randomised controlled trial (RCT) widely accepted as the gold standard. The RCT removes the effect of

the biases inherent in the early detection of disease by screening. It is, however, the most difficult type of study to conduct, and is often expensive and lengthy. Furthermore, an RCT can generally only address one principle outcome measure, such as lung cancer mortality, without being so large it becomes impractical to run. An alternative to the RCT is the population-based study, whereby the impact of a broadly implemented screening programme is assessed through changes in disease-specific mortality rates within the population. A third approach is the observational study with screening in selected cohorts, whereby the efficacy of the screening test is inferred from the frequency of detecting early-stage cancers.

## Methods of screening for lung cancer: evidence from clinical trials

The first English book on chest radiography was published in 1905. The initial chest films were of rather poor quality but enabled the drainage of a pneumothorax (collapsed lung) under X-ray control at Guys Hospital, London in 1907. It is now difficult to imagine the management of chest disease without the benefit of chest radiography. The chest X-ray (CXR) seemed to be the obvious method of screening individuals for lung cancer as it is a widely available, acceptable and relatively cheap test (Figures 10.1 and 10.2).

The first lung cancer screening studies began in the 1960s and by the 1980s there were around 10 major prospective screening studies using CXR and/or sputum cytology (i.e. checking phlegm under the microscope to find cancer cells), with over 300,000 individuals enrolled. Most excluded women; all included individuals over 45 years of age. Unfortunately most were not properly conducted randomised studies as both arms of the

---

*ABC of Lung Cancer*. Edited by I. Hunt, M. Muers and T. Treasure. © 2009 Blackwell Publishing, ISBN: 978-1-4051-4652-4.

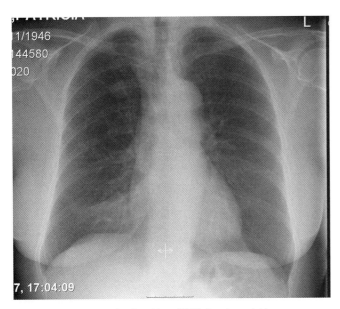

**Figure 10.1** An image of a chest X-ray (CXR) showing a right upper zone mass.

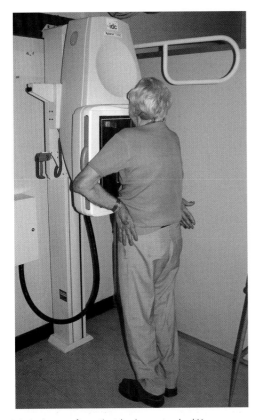

**Figure 10.2** An image of a patient having a standard X-ray.

Box 10.2 **Definitions of outcome measures**

$$\text{Mortality} = \frac{\text{Number of cancer deaths}}{\text{Number of patients screened}}$$

$$(\text{Mortality} = \text{Incidence} \times \text{Fatality})$$

$$\text{Fatality} = \frac{\text{Number of cancer deaths}}{\text{Number of cancers detected}}$$

Survival = Average length of time from diagnosis to death

remained true on follow-up for 20 years. Other methods of analysis for these studies have shown the screened patients to have a higher incidence of lung cancer, a higher rate of surgical resection and improved survival.

Much has been written about the methodology and findings of these studies in an attempt to explain why, despite an apparent improvement in survival in the screened group there was no reduction in lung cancer mortality. The outcome measured after screening influences the interpretation of any result and particularly the effect of screening biases. Measures such as survival and fatality are influenced, but mortality, especially cause-specific mortality is often held to be immune to the effects of such biases (Box 10.2). Furthermore, a comparison between screening-detected lung cancer and others detected by symptoms and signs appears to overestimate benefit because the former consists of cases that were diagnosed earlier, progress more slowly, and may never become clinically relevant. This comparison is therefore said to be biased. Lead-time, length and over diagnosis biases all appear to inflate the survival of screen-detected cases. Early diagnosis in screen-detected lung cancer patients falsely appears to prolong survival. However, the actual course of the disease ending in mortality is the same whether you screen or not (Figure 10.3a). Overestimation of survival duration among screening-detected lung cancer is caused by the relative excess of slowly progressing cases. Screening overrepresents less aggressive disease (Figure 10.3b) and detects 'biologically unimportant' tumours as well as those that are significant. This leads to an overestimation of survival duration among screen-detected cases caused by inclusion of 'subclinical' disease that would not become overt before the patient dies of other causes (Figure 10.3c). As a consequence of these studies, routine screening with CXR with or without sputum cytology is currently not recommended.

There has been a renewed interest in lung cancer screening in conjunction with the advent of modern CT scanners. Low-dose CT (LDCT), often referred to as 'spiral or helical' CT, is a technique that allows an image of the entire chest to be obtained in a single breath-hold with low radiation exposure (Figures 10.4 and 10.5).

Much of the evaluation of lung cancer screening with LDCT has come from observational studies, many of which were completed in Japan, a country that has had CT screening programmes running for over a decade. These studies have shown that LDCT can detect much smaller lung nodules than CXR and, as such, increase the ability to detect early-stage lung cancer.

studies allowed the use of CXR in asymptomatic patients. All reported lung cancer mortality as an outcome. The results from these studies showed no significant reduction in mortality in the screened population compared to the control arm. Importantly, the number of cases of lung cancers detected in the screened arm was higher than in the control arm, and for the study that was most thoroughly analysed – the Mayo Lung Project – this

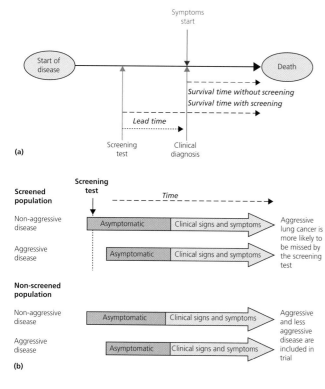

**(a)**

**(b)**

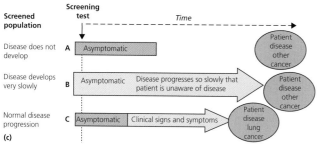

**(c)**

**Figure 10.3** Types of biases that can affect screening trials: (a) lead-time bias; (b) length bias; and (c) overdiagnosis bias. In (c) A and B are picked up by a screening test but otherwise would not be identified. Patients in examples A and B do not die of lung cancer and are likely to have a longer life expectancy. This leads to an over estimate of survival from the time of the screening test.

However, many lung nodules detected are not lung cancer, but rather are due to benign disease; this constitutes a false-positive screening test. These false positives have been shown to result in further tests, some of which may be invasive, and on occasion have resulted in thoracotomy for benign disease. Additionally, proof of the benefit of the detection of early-stage lung cancer using LDCT is not yet available.

The debate about the role of LDCT in lung cancer screening, particularly with continuing technological advances, remains intense. A number of large screening RCT comparing 'spiral' CT against conventional CXR are currently underway and their results are awaited with much interest. In addition, protocols have been developed in how to manage patients with solitary pulmonary nodules so as to improve the accuracy of diagnosis and to reduce overinvestigation or useless intervention (Figure 10.6). Currently, however, there is no evidence to support the use of LDCT in screening for lung cancer and no international lung cancer guideline has recommended its adoption.

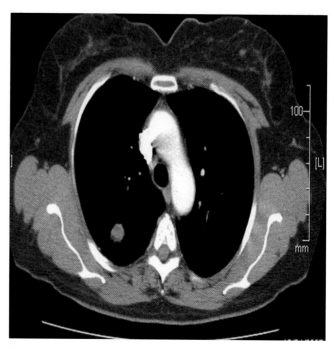

**Figure 10.4** A computed tomography (CT) image demonstrating a solitary pulmonary nodule.

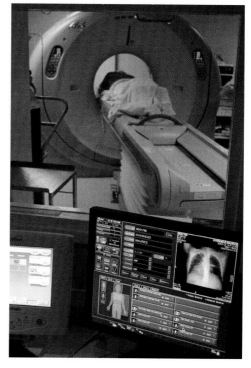

**Figure 10.5** An image of a modern computed tomography (CT) machine in use.

## The future of lung cancer screening

With an increasing number of biomarkers being identified, early detection of lung cancer or even premalignant lesions through a non-radiological approach appears increasingly feasible. Various candidate biomarkers are currently under evaluation and include markers of genetic, histological and phenotypic tissue changes

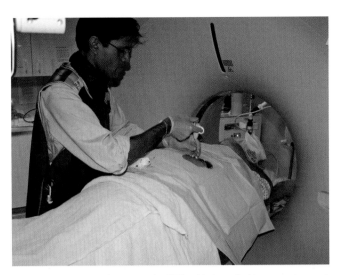

**Figure 10.6** Computed tomography (CT)-guided needle biopsy can be used to obtain histological proof of diagnosis in suspicious nodules that are large enough to biopsy.

associated with the process of carcinogenesis. Most of these new methods involve screening by obtaining cells of the bronchial epithelia, as biopsies or brushings, from sputum or through blood samples. So far the most successful approach for obtaining appropriate specimens is through bronchoscopy, though clearly peripheral blood testing would be a preferred method of screening. Such biomarker tests currently remain research tools only.

The original RCT for screening lung cancer using the CXR and/or sputum cytology lung cancer were generally regarded as showing no benefit. The current randomised LDCT screening trials will show whether modern technology confers a genuine benefit to patients, or simply detects smaller biologically unimportant disease.

## Further reading

Alberts WM. Diagnosis and management of lung cancer executive summary: ACCP evidence-based clinical practice guidelines (2nd Edition). *Chest* 2007; **132**(Suppl 3): 1S–19.

Manser RL, Irving L, Byrnes G, Abramson M, Stone C & Campbell D. Screening for lung cancer: a systematic review and meta-analysis of controlled trial. *Thorax* 2003; **58**: 784–789.

Treasure T, Hunt I, Keogh B & Pagano D, eds. *The Evidence for Cardiothoracic Surgery*. tfm publishing, Shrewsbury, 2004.

International Early Lung Cancer Action Project (ELCAP) (http://www.ielcap.org)

# CHAPTER 11

# Supportive and Palliative Care

*Andrew Wilcock, Richard Neal and Patricia Hunt*

---

**OVERVIEW**

- Supportive care refers to treatments used to reduce or eliminate symptoms from cancer and/or treatment side-effects.
- Palliative care is similar but refers to symptom management and special care of a person whose disease cannot be cured.
- Both share the common aim of providing the best possible quality of life by maximizing the patient's comfort and minimizing their suffering.
- Good communication skills and a multidisciplinary approach are prerequisites for successful physical, psychological, social and spiritual care.
- Specialist palliative care services should become involved when distressing symptoms are unrelieved and/or when there are complex psychosocial or spiritual issues.

---

Nine out of ten patients presenting with lung cancer die of it and many within a year of diagnosis. Thus, supportive care (alongside oncological treatment) and palliative care (when life-prolonging measures are no longer possible or become counter-productive) are important. The primary and secondary healthcare teams mainly provide such care, supported as necessary by other specialists and palliative care services. In addition to physical symptoms (Box 11.1), the psychological, social and spiritual aspects of suffering must be addressed.

Lung cancer is a disease of the elderly, tends to affect the more deprived, and is at risk of being stigmatised as being self-inflicted. Compared to other cancers there are diagnostic delays and communication in hospital is believed to be poorer, partly due to difficulty with the socio-demographic group and partly due to the complex nature of the messages that have to be relayed.

## A general approach to symptom management

A structured approach to symptom management is encapsulated in the acronym 'EEMMA', developed by Twycross and Wilcock in 2001 (see Box 11.2).

---

*ABC of Lung Cancer.* Edited by I. Hunt, M. Muers and T. Treasure. © 2009 Blackwell Publishing, ISBN: 978-1-4051-4652-4.

---

Box 11.1 **Common symptoms of lung cancer**

- Fatigue
- Pain, e.g. chest, bone
- Anorexia-cachexia
- Cough
- Breathlessness
- Insomnia
- Haemoptysis
- Hoarse voice
- Nausea and vomiting (in those receiving chemotherapy)
- Alopecia (in those receiving radiotherapy)
- Dysphagia (in those receiving radiotherapy)
- Sore throat (in those receiving radiotherapy)

---

Box 11.2 **Approaching symptom management (EEMMA)**
**(Reproduced with permission from Twycross & Wilcock 2001)**

- **Evaluation**: of the impact of the illness on the patient and family, and of the causes of the patient's symptoms (often multifactorial).
- **Explanation**: to the patient before starting treatment about what is going on, and discussion on what is the most appropriate course of action.
- **Management**: correct the correctable, non-drug treatment or drug treatment.
- **Monitoring**: frequent review of the impact of treatment; optimising the doses of symptom relief drugs to maximise benefit and minimise undesirable effects.
- **Attention to detail**: do not make unwarranted assumptions; listen actively to the patient, respond to non-verbal and verbal cues.

## Management of common symptoms

### Breathlessness

*Correct the correctable*: includes oncological treatments such as chemotherapy, radiotherapy, surgical, laser, photodynamic or cryosurgical debulking of tumours obstructing large airways, and supportive therapies such as blood transfusion for anaemia and endoluminal stenting for compression of a large airway (Figure 11.1).

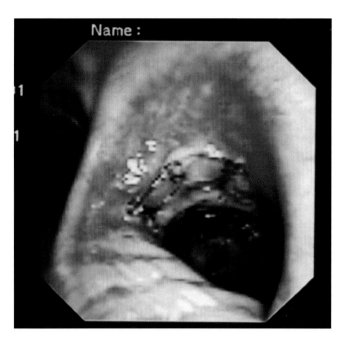

**Figure 11.1** An illustration of an endobronchial stent.

Box 11.3 **Use of morphine for breathlessness at rest**

**In opioid-naïve patients:**
- start with small doses of morphine, e.g. 2.5–5 mg orally, as required; larger doses can be poorly tolerated;
- if ≥2 doses/24 h are needed, prescribe morphine regularly and titrate the dose according to response, duration of effect and undesirable side-effects; and
- relatively small doses may suffice, e.g. 20–60 mg/24 h.

**In patients already taking morphine for pain and with:**
- severe breathlessness (i.e. ≥7/10), a dose that is 100% or more of the 5-times daily analgesic dose may be needed;
- moderate breathlessness (i.e. 4–6/10), a dose equivalent to 50–100% of the 5-times daily analgesic dose may suffice; or
- mild breathlessness (i.e. ≤3/10), a dose equivalent to 25–50% of the 5-times daily analgesic dose may suffice.

In some patients, diamorphine/morphine by continuous subcutaneous infusion is better tolerated and provides greater relief, possibly by avoiding the peaks (with undesirable effects) and troughs (with loss of effect) of oral medication.

Doses are a guide only: prescribers should consult the *British National Formulary*.

*Non-drug treatment*: includes the use of an electric fan, relaxation therapies and techniques that re-enforce efficient breathing (emphasising expiration and activity pacing). Patients often fear suffocating to death, and prophylactic discussion with them and their family about the relief of terminal breathlessness is important.

*Drug treatment*: severe breathlessness is frightening and often triggers episodes of respiratory panic. These should be enquired about, discussed and, if necessary, treated with anxiolytics (short-term) and/or a selective serotonin reuptake inhibitor (SSRI; long-term). It is also important not to miss concurrent depression that generally responds to specific treatment. Morphine reduces the ventilatory response to hypercapnoea, hypoxia and exercise, thus decreasing respiratory effort and breathlessness. Improvements are seen at doses that do not cause respiratory depression. Clinical trial evidence supports the use of opioids by the oral and parenteral (intravenous) but not the nebulised route. Generally opioids are more beneficial for breathlessness at rest rather than upon exertion. Even with maximal exertion, breathlessness generally recovers within a few minutes, and non-drug approaches should be used. The combination of an opioid and a sedative anxiolytic, such as midazolam, given subcutaneously by syringe driver may be necessary terminally (Box 11.3).

## Cough

*Correct the correctable*: such as radiotherapy for the primary cancer.

*Non-drug treatment*: includes advice about how to cough efficiently, physiotherapy and steam inhalations.

*Drug treatment*: includes the appropriate use of protussives (expectorants) for a productive cough, and antitussives for a dry cough. Codeine is a useful antitussive but, if ineffective, it should be replaced by morphine.

## Weight loss and fatigue

Although many symptoms such as weight loss (cachexia), loss of appetite (anorexia), and fatigue are common, there is little strong evidence to guide management. Benefit may well come from a multidisciplinary approach, including a dietician and the use of dietary supplements, an occupational therapist and a physiotherapist. Cachexia-anorexia syndrome may be associated with a chronic inflammatory state induced by the cancer rather than the cancer itself. Awareness of this might direct attention to other and better management strategies.

## Palliative interventions for lung cancer

Although strong evidence is sparse or non-existent for many symptom treatments, there is still much that can be done. Patients whose symptoms do not readily respond to standard measures should be referred without delay for specialist palliative care.

### Pleural effusion

Drainage of pleural effusion often eases the associated breathlessness and cough. Drainage is performed through a small-bore chest tube and, when the lung has completely re-expanded, it can be followed up with a talc pleurodesis. Rolling and tipping the supine patient in an attempt to distribute the talc is unnecessary. However, thoracoscopic pleurodesis (medical or surgical) may be more effective than tube pleurodesis.

### Superior vena cava obstruction

A right-sided lung cancer or the presence of mediastinal lymph nodes can lead to compression of the superior vena cava (SVC), causing oedema of the face, neck and arms, with or without distended veins over the chest. The obstruction can be exacerbated by thrombosis.

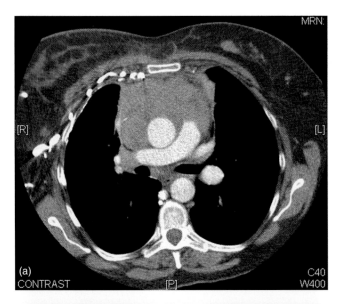

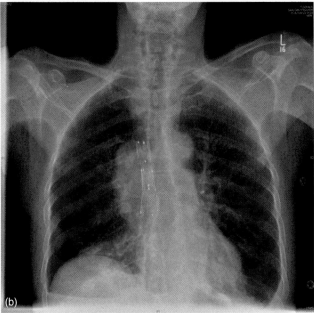

Figure 11.2 An illustration of a superior vena cava (SVC) stent.

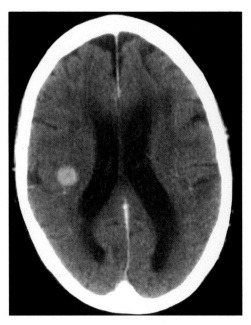

Figure 11.3 An illustration of a brain metastasis on a computed tomography (CT) scan.

A corticosteroid such as dexamethasone is traditionally given on diagnosis, followed by chemotherapy (generally for small-cell lung cancer, SCLC) and/or radiotherapy (generally for non-small cell lung cancer, NSCLC). A self-expanding stent placed percutaneously into the SVC provides immediate relief (Figure 11.2).

## Brain metastases

Brain metastases occur frequently in patients with lung cancer, especially SCLC. They may present with headaches, limb weakness, epileptic seizures, cognitive impairment and/or lethargy (Figure 11.3). Corticosteroids are effective in the short-term, but undesirable side-effects are common. The median survival is one to two months with corticosteroids alone, but four months if combined with whole-brain radiotherapy; chemotherapy may also be beneficial. Surgical resection of a solitary brain metastasis should be limited to patients with NSCLC who have had a complete resection of the primary tumour and have no other metastatic disease.

## Spinal cord compression

Compression of the spinal cord by metastases causes variable neurological impairment, including paraplegia (Figure 11.4). Common presenting symptoms are pain, weakness, autonomic dysfunction and sensory loss. The aim is to make the diagnosis before gross (generally irreversible) neurological abnormalities are present. Thus practitioners require a high index of suspicion, particularly in high-risk patients, for example SCLC and thoracic spine metastases, and when there are symptoms suggestive of early cord compression. Patients with spinal cord compression should be treated within 24 hours with corticosteroids and radiotherapy, and also surgery if appropriate.

## Hypercalcaemia and bone pain

An intravenous bisphosphonate is the treatment of choice for hypercalcemia of malignancy. Bone metastases are common in lung cancer, presenting either as pain or as pathological fracture (Figure 11.5). Management includes the use of analgesics, radiotherapy, bisphosphonates and occasionally nerve blocks. A single radiotherapy treatment is often sufficient. Most patients benefit within one to two weeks, but it can take more than four weeks. The median duration of relief is 12 weeks.

## Psychological aspects of terminal illness

Downturns in a patient's emotions are common and tend to be most marked at the time of diagnosis, at the time of first recurrence, and as death approaches. Up to 15% of people with advanced cancer have an identifiable depressive illness.

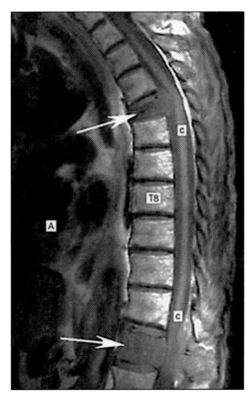

**Figure 11.4** Magnetic resonance imaging (MRI) of the spine showing spinal cord compression.

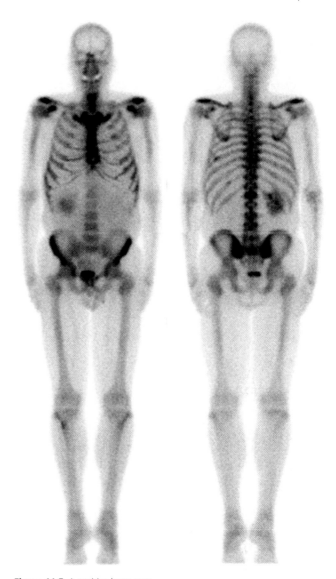

**Figure 11.5** A positive bone scan.

Psychological distress is also common among relatives. Unfortunately, much of the psychological distress of both the patient and their relatives remains undetected. Screening for such distress at diagnosis and beyond may detect significant psychosocial problems that, if addressed expediously and appropriately, may improve quality of life (Table 11.1).

Some psychological problems can be prevented by:
- good staff-patient communication, giving information according to individual need;
- good staff-patient relationships, with continuity of care; and
- giving people some control over the management of their illness.

Many people have a combination of good inner resources and good external support that enables them to cope without prolonged disabling distress. However, some people need specialist psychological intervention.

## Care of the relatives

Because relatives are often reluctant to bother busy health professionals, communication between the relatives and the team should be initiated and maintained proactively. Involving the patient together with their family from the start prevents collusion and a conspiracy of silence. However, opportunity should also be provided for seeing both the patient and the close family separately, whilst being aware of important issues of confidentiality, in case of a reluctance to ask certain questions in the other's presence.

## Spiritual care

Spirituality is the valuing of the non-material aspects of life, including the transcendent. It is concerned with achieving harmony with both the world within and the world around, and thus strives for answers about personal meaning in life and about God, including the meaning of suffering and death. For people with advanced disease there is often an increased need for acceptance and affirmation by those around them, and for forgiveness and reconciliation with family and friends. In this respect, a practitioner's primary responsibility is to help maintain an environment that is supportive of the patient. Some intractable symptoms may reflect unexpressed spiritual distress and specific enquiry may be necessary. Remember that those who accept a specific religious label are often not orthodox in their beliefs. Thus, always listen to the patient and do not make unwarranted assumptions.

**Table 11.1** Common psychological responses to loss

| Phase | Symptoms | Typical duration |
|---|---|---|
| Disruption | Disbelief<br>Denial<br>Shock/numbness<br>Despair | Days–weeks |
| Dysphoria | Anxiety<br>Insomnia<br>Poor concentration<br>Anger<br>Guilt<br>Activities disrupted<br>Sadness<br>Depression | Weeks–months |
| Adaptation | (as dysphoria diminishes)<br>Implications confronted<br>New goals established<br>Hope refocused and<br>restored<br>Activities resumed | Months–years |

Box 11.4 **The Gold Standards Framework (GSF)**

The GSF is a framework to enable a gold standard of care for all people nearing the end of their lives (http://www.goldstandardsframework.nhs.uk).

The seven 'gold' standards:
- Communication
- Coordination
- Control of symptoms
- Continuity out-of-hours
- Continued learning
- Carer support
- Care in the dying phase

Guidance for best practice on:
- Teamwork and continuity of care
- Advanced planning
- Symptom control
- Support of patients/carers

## Specific issues for primary care management

Many issues relating to the delivery of high-quality palliative and supportive care are generic to all sectors within the health service. However, much palliative and supportive care is provided by primary care, which often has specific needs. General practitioners ideally need to work closely with local teams, and to seek their specialist advice where appropriate. The gold standards pathway focuses on improving clinical and organisational knowledge and the human dimension of service delivery. It is based on seven 'gold' standards to encourage and enable practices to improve care for patients approaching the end of their lives (and is published by the NHS) (see Box 11.4).

## Last days of life

As part of a national quality improvement initiative, the use of the Liverpool Care of the Dying Pathway is being encouraged. It is intended for patients in the last few days of life and facilitates a change in focus from life-preservation to comfort-in-dying. When the pathway is applied to individual patients a standard protocol is used. This includes a checklist of things to be considered, such as reviewing long-term medication, whether intravenous hydration is still appropriate, and a reminder to discuss the changing situation with the patient's family, as well as guidelines on the management of common symptoms, such as pain, breathlessness, vomiting and delirium. People with lung cancer and their families have a right to high-quality holistic, supportive and palliative care.

## Acknowledgement

We would like to thank Dr Robert Twycross for his helpful comments.

## Further reading

Ahmedzai SH & Muers MF. *Supportive Care in Respiratory Disease*. Oxford University Press, Oxford, 2005.

Booth S & Dudgeon D. *Dyspnoea in Advanced Disease*. Oxford University Press, Oxford, 2006.

Ellershaw J & Wilkinson S. *Care of the Dying. A Pathway to Excellence*. Oxford University Press, Oxford, 2003. See also http://www.lcp-mariecurie.org.uk.

National Audit Office. *Tackling Cancer: Improving the Patient Journey*. National Audit Office, London, 2005.

The Gold Standards Pathway: http://www.goldstandardsframework.nhs.uk.

NICE. *Guidance on Cancer Services: Improving Supportive and Palliative Care for Adults with Cancer – the Manual*. National Institute for Health & Clinical Excellence, London, 2004: http://www.nice.org.uk.

SIGN. *Control of Pain in Patients with Cancer: A National Clinical Guideline*. Edinburgh: Scottish Intercollegiate Guidelines Network, 2000. http://www.sign.ac.uk.

Twycross R & Wilcock A. *Symptom Management in Advanced Cancer*, 3rd edition. Radcliffe Medical Press Limited, Oxford, 2001.

Twycross R & Wilcock A, eds. *Palliative Care Formulary*, 3rd edition. Palliativedrugs.com Ltd, Nottingham, 2007. See also http://www.palliative-drugs.com.

Wilcock A & Twycross, R. Symptom management in palliative care: optimizing drug treatment. *British Journal of Hospital Medicine* 2006; **67**(8): 400–403.

# Index

*Note:* Page numbers in *italics* refer to figures, those in **bold** refer to tables and boxes

**53**